NUTRITIONAL SCREENING AND ASSESSMENT TOOLS

NUTRITIONAL SCREENING AND ASSESSMENT TOOLS

J. M. JONES

Nova Science Publishers, Inc.
New York

Copyright © 2006 by Nova Science Publishers, Inc.

All rights reserved. No part of this book may be reproduced, stored in a retrieval system or transmitted in any form or by any means: electronic, electrostatic, magnetic, tape, mechanical photocopying, recording or otherwise without the written permission of the Publisher.

For permission to use material from this book please contact us:
Telephone 631-231-7269; Fax 631-231-8175
Web Site: http://www.novapublishers.com

NOTICE TO THE READER
The Publisher has taken reasonable care in the preparation of this book, but makes no expressed or implied warranty of any kind and assumes no responsibility for any errors or omissions. No liability is assumed for incidental or consequential damages in connection with or arising out of information contained in this book. The Publisher shall not be liable for any special, consequential, or exemplary damages resulting, in whole or in part, from the readers' use of, or reliance upon, this material.

Independent verification should be sought for any data, advice or recommendations contained in this book. In addition, no responsibility is assumed by the publisher for any injury and/or damage to persons or property arising from any methods, products, instructions, ideas or otherwise contained in this publication.

This publication is designed to provide accurate and authoritative information with regard to the subject matter cover herein. It is sold with the clear understanding that the Publisher is not engaged in rendering legal or any other professional services. If legal, medical or any other expert assistance is required, the services of a competent person should be sought. FROM A DECLARATION OF PARTICIPANTS JOINTLY ADOPTED BY A COMMITTEE OF THE AMERICAN BAR ASSOCIATION AND A COMMITTEE OF PUBLISHERS.

Library of Congress Cataloging-in-Publication Data
Jones, J. M. (Jeanne Mary), 1956-
Nutritional screening and assessment tools / J.M. Jones.
    p. ; cm.
Includes index.
ISBN 1-59454-613-4
1. Nutrition--Evaluation. 2. Malnutrition--Diagnosis.
[DNLM: 1. Nutrition Assessment. 2. Malnutrition--diagnosis. 3. Mass Screening--methods. 4. Multivariate Analysis. QU 146.1 J77n 2005] I. Title.
RC621.J66   2005
363.8'63--dc22   2005022726

Published by Nova Science Publishers, Inc. ✢ New York

CONTENTS

Preface		vii
Introduction		ix
Chapter 1	Literature Search of Published Tools	1
Chapter 2	Selection of an Appropriate Tool	5
Chapter 3	Multivariate Analysis	23
Chapter 4	Reliability	33
Chapter 5	Validity	55
Chapter 6	Further Application of Findings	87
Conclusion		91
References		93
Index		101

PREFACE

Malnutrition is a serious problem amongst many sections of the population. Increases in morbidity and mortality, length of hospital stay and hence, cost of providing health care have all been attributable to this, so the identification of subjects at risk of malnutrition is essential to provide optimal nutrition during treatment and recovery. Many screening tools have been developed for the purpose of identifying subjects who are at risk of malnutrition. However, selection of the most appropriate instrument for use in a particular population is hampered by the sheer number of existing tools and the fact that many of these have not been rigorously developed and evaluated.

The aim of this book is to present guidelines and criteria to assist a practitioner to assess the scientific merit of nutritional screening and assessment tools using principles of sound design and analysis. The appraisal includes an assessment of the details regarding a tool's intended application, the methods used to derive the tool, and an evaluation of its performance. These features of a tool are considered under the headings of application, development and evaluation.

Specific criteria for assessing the quality of a tool and their rationale are presented within each section, together with the results of applying these standards to published tools. Shortcomings identified by this review are highlighted and the relevant methodology presented to help ensure that future studies are implemented with regard to these important research principles. An approach for tool development using a multivariate technique is outlined. Assessment of tool evaluation includes independence of measurements, use of appropriate administrators, adequate sample size, and correct methods of analysis. SPSS routines for sample size determination for reliability and validity studies are included.

Each stage of the process is illustrated with practical suggestions and examples, and concepts explained with the non-statistician in mind. Throughout the book, suggestions are made to guide a practitioner as to the application of these findings.

J. M. Jones[*]
Senior Lecturer in Medical Statistics, Mathematics Department,
Keele University, Keele, Staffordshire

---

[*] Dr. J.M. Jones, Senior Lecturer in Medical Statistics, Mathematics Department, Keele University, Keele, Staffordshire,ST5 5BG, UK. E-mail: j.m.jones@maths.keele.ac.uk

INTRODUCTION

The existence of malnutrition amongst many sections of the population is well documented. The finding [1] that approximately 40% of UK adult hospital patients are either malnourished or at high risk of malnutrition and that nutritional status often worsens following admission, indicates how serious a problem malnutrition is to the provision of proper medical care. Increases in morbidity and mortality, length of hospital stay and hence, cost of providing health care have all been attributable to this [2-4]. Hence, the identification of subjects at risk of malnutrition is essential to provide optimal nutrition during treatment and recovery [3,5]. Although malnutrition encompasses both under-nutrition and over-nutrition, this book focuses only on under-nutrition.

The introduction of routine nutritional risk screening has been hindered by the lack of a widely accepted screening system which would detect patients who might benefit from nutritional support. It is only recently, that guidelines for nutrition risk screening, applicable to different settings (community, hospital, elderly care), have been proposed [6].

The success of any screening programme depends on using the right tool for the job. Many screening tools have been developed for the purpose of identifying subjects who are malnourished or at risk of malnutrition. These tools are usually presented as a questionnaire or proforma, comprising variables associated with malnutrition, and a subject's nutritional status or malnutrition risk is determined based on responses to these risk factors.

The production of nutritional screening or assessment tools has been likened to that of a 'cottage industry' [7], with many hospitals, groups or individuals deriving their own tool. The resultant plethora of nutritional tools makes it difficult to select the most appropriate for use in a particular clinical environment [8]. Moreover, there is an increasing realisation that many published tools have not been carefully evaluated [9-12], and hence cannot be relied on to provide an accurate diagnosis or offer guidance for providing appropriate care and support [8].

How should practitioners find their way through this maze to locate the 'best' tool to aid in the nutritional evaluation of a particular subject population? The aim of this book is to present guidelines and criteria to assist in the identification of a suitable instrument. Criteria by which their relative merits may be judged include practical and methodological issues. Practical considerations may include availability of a tool which is easy to understand, and is simple and quick to use. Methodological criteria require evidence of its performance and effectiveness.

The book presents a critical appraisal of published instruments using principles of sound design and analysis, and considers the methodology behind the development and evaluation of nutritional screening and assessment tools. Each stage of the process is illustrated with practical suggestions and examples, and concepts explained with the non-statistician in mind. Suggestions are made to guide a practitioner as to the use or application of these research findings.

Lyne and Prowse [11] highlighted the lack of clarity concerning the definitions of nutritional terms, in particular 'nutritional assessment' and 'nutritional screening'. They concluded that the desired outcome of assessment is to measure actual nutritional status in clinically meaningful terms, whereas the desired outcome of screening is to estimate the degree of exposure to risk of nutritional compromise. It is essential to be very clear about the purpose of using any tool. However, consideration of the statistical aspects of tool development and evaluation does not require a distinction to be made between tools for assessment and tools for screening because they share the same methodological issues. These instruments may differ in the type and nature of the information collected, but they have the common purpose of using all or some of this data to obtain the relevant outcome for a subject, that is, nutritional status for an assessment tool and risk of malnutrition for a screening tool. This book refers to all such instruments using the term 'nutritional tools'.

Chapter 1

LITERATURE SEARCH OF PUBLISHED TOOLS

In 2000, a systematic search of published literature was undertaken using clearly defined criteria to assemble an array of nutritional tools [13]. Studies identified by the search were published within the previous 25 years. The purpose of these papers was classified into the following four groups:

- presentation of an original nutritional screening or assessment tool
- evaluation of an existing tool in a different population to the one for which it was initially developed
- presentation of a modified version of an existing nutritional tool
- use of an existing tool to estimate the prevalence of malnutrition in a group of people under study.

For the purpose of appraising the methodology behind the development and evaluation of nutritional tools, the fourth kind of study was not relevant and hence such studies were not considered further. Multi-stage screening studies, in which at each screen a different questionnaire is used by a different professional group, were also excluded from the review in order to concentrate on the evaluation of a single nutritional tool for each study reviewed.

The literature search identified 44 instruments with an outcome variable associated with nutritional status or risk of malnutrition. Each tool was classified according to the population of subjects for which it was intended. Thirty two studies presented an original tool and are listed in Table 1(a). Twenty three of these studies considered a tool for use amongst hospital inpatients, one study assessed nutritional status in an out-patient setting, and eight studies developed a tool for use in the community or long-stay hospital.

The 12 studies (Table 1(b)) that either evaluated an existing tool in a new population, or modified an existing instrument are considered separately from those that presented an original tool because some of the methodological issues applicable to the development of an original tool may not apply. Eight of the 12 studies were carried out amongst in-patients, two amongst out-patients and two used a tool in the community or nursing home. The version of the Subjective Global Assessment tool [44] used by Detsky *et al.* [53] was used unmodified in three studies [48,50,54] and modified versions were evaluated by four studies [47,49,55,56]. Hickson and Hill [46] adapted the Nutrition Risk Score [23] for use in the community.

This tool was also used by Wright [52], who made a minor modification to the categories of body mass index. Prendergast *et al.* [51] used the Nutritional Risk Index [19] in an out-patient setting, and the tool developed by Potosnak *et al.* [34] was further evaluated by Brown and Stegman [57].

It was evident from this literature search that a considerable amount of time and effort have been expended on developing tools to assist in the diagnosis of malnutrition. Some were developed because no relevant tool existed for the subjects under assessment [17,32,33], or because existing tools were not practical [25,42], or to derive a generic tool which was simple, quick, reliable and valid [21,22]. It is likely that many other nutritional screening and assessment tools exist besides those considered in this review, with hospitals using their own in-house unpublished technique [58].

Table 1(a). Studies that presented an original nutritional tool

Population	Tool	Lead Author [Reference]
Children with Special Health Care Needs	Nutrition Screening Form	Clark [14]
	PEACH Survey	Campbell [15]
Community Patients	Community Focused Nutrition Screening Tool	Gilford [16]
	Nutritional Risk Assessment Tool	Ward [17]
Elderly Subjects	Mini Nutritional Assessment	Guigoz [18]
	Nutritional Risk Index	Wolinsky [19]
Hospital Patients	Admission Nutrition Screening Tool	Kovacevich [20]
Adult	Derby Nutritional Score	Goudge [21]
	Malnutrition Screening Tool	Ferguson [22]
Hospital Patients	Nutrition Risk Score	Reilly [23]
Adult + Paediatric	Nutrition Screening Card	Nagel [24]
	Screening Nutritional Profile	Hunt [25]
Hospital Patients	Nutrition Screening Form	Hedberg [26]
Age not stated	Nutrition Status Algorithm	Lowery [27]
Hospital Patients	Nursing Nutrition Screening Assessment	Pattison [28]
Elderly	Nursing Nutritional Screening Tool	Cotton [29]
	Nutritional Risk Assessment Scale	Nikolaus [30]
Juvenile Rheumatoid Arthritis	Nutritional Screening Test	Henderson [31]
Learning Difficulties	Nutrition Screening Form	Bryan [32]
Long-term Care Residents	Nutrition Screening Tool	Noel [33]
Medical and Surgical	East Orange Nutritional Screening Form	Potosnak [34]
	Nutrition Assessment Score	Oakley [35]
	Nutrition Screening Equation	Elmore [36]

Table 1(a). Studies that presented an original nutritional tool

Population	Tool	Lead Author [Reference]
Oncology	Nutritional Screen Form	Lundvick [37]
	Oncology Screening Tools	Latkany [38]
Oral and Maxillofacial Malignancy	General Nutritional Status Score	Guo [39]
Surgical	Clinical Assessment	Hall [40]
	Clinical Judgement	Lupo [41]
	Nursing Nutritional Assessment Tool	Scanlan [42]
	Nutritional Screening	Thompson [43]
	Subjective Global Assessment (SGA)	Baker [44]
Trauma	Nutrition Checklist	Cooper [45]

Table 1(b). Studies that evaluated an existing or modified nutritional tool

Population	Tool (Originator)	Lead Author [Reference]
Community	Nutrition Risk Score (Reilly [23])	Hickson [46]
Dialysis	Dialysis Malnutrition Score (Detsky [53])	Kalantar-Zadeh [47]
	Subjective Global Assessment (Detsky [53])	Enia [48]
	7 Point SGA scale (Detsky [53])	Visser [49]
Elderly		
Inpatients	Subjective Global Assessment (Detsky [53])	Ek [50]
Male outpatients	Nutritional Risk Index (Wolinsky [19])	Prendergast [51]
Nursing or residential homes	Nutrition Risk Score (Hickson [46])	Wright [52]
Gastroenterology	Subjective Global Assessment (Baker [44])	Detsky [53]
	Subjective Global Assessment (Detsky [53])	Hirsch [54]
HIV Infected	Revised SGA (Detsky [53])	Bowers [55]
Liver Transplant	Subjective Nutrition Assessment Tool (Detsky [53])	Hasse [56]
Medical and Surgical	East Orange Nutritional Screening Form (Potosnak [34])	Brown [57]

Chapter 2

SELECTION OF AN APPROPRIATE TOOL

Let us suppose we wish to identify an appropriate tool for assessing the nutritional status or risk of malnutrition of a defined subject population. Figure 1 outlines the various stages involved in this process.

The first step should always be a search of the literature in order to determine potentially relevant tools which have been developed for the specific patient group of interest. Having identified such tools, we then need to judge their relevance, usefulness, scientific merit, and evidence base by considering their practicalities and methodological issues.

Practical considerations may vary according to the context in which the tool will be used, but are likely to include the availability of a tool that uses information that is feasible to collect, is presented in a format that is clear and simple to follow, and allows a nutritional evaluation to be carried out within an achievable time scale [59]. A clearly described action plan, presence of a manual or required training needs of administrators, and incorporation of the tool into existing procedures will also be of benefit to potential users.

Methodological appraisal of a tool covers three stages. Firstly, we need to check the intended application of a tool is suitable for our needs. Secondly, we need to be confident that the tool has been developed using an appropriate method and is based on factors known to be associated with malnutrition. Thirdly, we require evidence that the tool performs well. These three features can be termed application, development and evaluation, respectively.

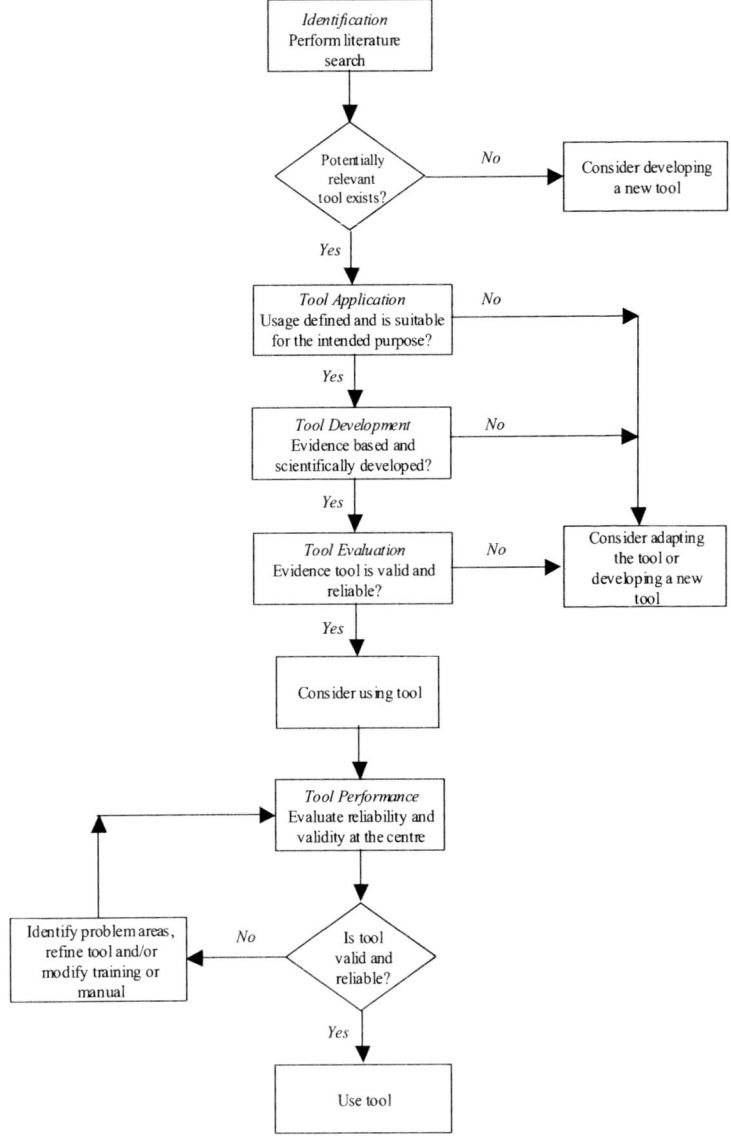

Figure 1. Flowchart depicting the selection of an appropriate tool

The structure of this book is to consider each of these three aspects separately. Criteria for evaluating each aspect are detailed, and used to assess the scientific merit of the published tools listed in Tables 1(a) and 1(b). The resultant critical appraisal considers more features and provides additional detailed descriptions of tool methodology than it was possible to include in the original review [13]. Shortcomings identified by the review are highlighted and the relevant methodology presented. The methods presented have been selected on the grounds of simplicity. They may not necessarily give an optimal design or most efficient analysis, but are considered preferable due to their relative ease of implementation.

A. TOOL APPLICATION

For a tool to be of benefit to potential users, it must be published with sufficient information to allow correct usage [13]. Criteria to assess this are listed in Table 2. These include a definition of the population for which the tool is intended, specifying inclusion and exclusion criteria. The outcome variable and associated risk groups should also be defined. The time-points during a subject's care at which the tool should be used, and its intended administrator(s) are also prerequisites to appropriate tool usage.

Each paper identified by the literature search was searched for the presence of this information. If a recommended time of usage was not stated but the study described its experience with the tool, then the study application time was assumed to be the recommended time. Tables 3(a) and 3(b), respectively, present the application details for each new tool, and for those that were either evaluated in a new population or were modifications of an existing tool.

Table 2. Criteria for assessing a nutritional tool: Application

TOOL APPLICATION
Definitions of:
Target population
Outcome variable and risk groups
Initial and subsequent times of administration
Professional group(s) of administrators

Target Population

All papers documented the population for which the tool was designed, although some developed for use in acute care failed to give an age range.

Outcome Variable and Risk Groups

Definition of the outcome variable was a prerequisite for inclusion in the review. The associated nutritional risk groups were not defined by one study [47]. No tool had more than four risk groups. Fifteen (47%) of the 32 original tools had two groups, eleven (34%) had three and six (19%) had four risk groups. Nine of the 12 studies that evaluated or modified an existing instrument used a tool with three categories. Each risk group should be linked to a clear plan of action, whether this is to encourage greater food consumption, offer fortified meals, refer to a dietitian, instigate nutritional support or offer regular monitoring of nutritional status [6,8], but only a few studies gave detailed action plans. These were primarily published for tools administered by nursing staff [21,29,42,45,46,52].

Initial and Subsequent Times of Administration

Twenty six (81%) of the 32 original tools and ten (83%) of the 12 studies that evaluated or modified an existing tool gave the initial time of screening or assessment. However a precise definition of this time-point was not always stated; in particular, several of the tools for hospital in-patients merely described this as 'on admission'. Although reassessment should form part of the pathway for provision of nutritional support [60,61], with frequency dependent upon the specific population [61,62], only thirteen (41%) of the new tools and four (33%) of the existing or modified tools considered this. Precise definitions of the time-points or situations during a patient's care at which reassessment should be carried out were also often omitted.

Table 3(a). Studies that presented an original nutritional tool: Outcome variable, time of assessment and administrator

Population	Lead Author [Reference]	Outcome Variable	Time of Assessment	Intended Administrator
Children with Special Health Care Needs	Clark [14]	Recommend nutritionist referral: yes, no	Not specified; re-screen at regular intervals	Early intervention team members
	Campbell [15]	Probable nutrition problem: yes, no	Not specified	Primary caregiver
Community patients	Gilford [16]	Malnutrition risk: low, moderate, high	Not specified	Community nurse
	Ward [17]	Undernutrition risk: none, possible or probable, malnourished	Not specified; reassess regularly	Primary health care team member
Elderly Subjects	Guigoz [18]	Nutritional status: well nourished, at risk, malnourished	On admission to hospital or nursing home; part of a geriatric assessment programme	Health professional at hospital or nursing home, general physician
	Wolinsky [19]	Nutritional risk: high, low	Not specified	Relatively untrained and unskilled personnel
Hospital Patients Adult	Kovacevich [20]	Nutritional risk: low, at risk	Within 48 hours of admission	Nurse
	Goudge [21]	Nutritional risk: yes, no	On admission	Nurse
	Ferguson [22]	Malnutrition risk: yes, no	Within 24 hours of admission and re-screen weekly	Medical, nursing, dietetic, admin staff, family, friends, patients
Hospital Patients Adult + Paediatric	Reilly [23]	Nutrition risk: low, moderate, high	On admission and repeat weekly	Nurse
	Nagel [24]	Nutritional risk: low, moderate, high	Within 48/72 hours of admission and re-screen in 4/7 days	Nutrition assistant, dietitian
	Hunt [25]	Malnutrition risk: low, high	Within 24 hours of admission	Patient, nurse and dietetic technician complete the form

Table 3(a). Continued

Population	Lead Author [Reference]	Outcome Variable	Time of Assessment	Intended Administrator
Hospital Patients Age not stated	Hedberg [26]	Nutritional risk: yes, no	5th hospital day	Dietetic technician
	Lowery [27]	Nutrition status: normal, mildly, moderately, severely compromised	On admission	Dietitian, dietetic technician
Hospital Patients Elderly	Pattison [28]	Undernutrition risk: minimal, moderate, high	On admission and repeat weekly	Dietitian, nurse
	Cotton [29]	Undernutrition risk: minimal, moderate, high	Within 24 hours of admission and repeat weekly	Nurse
	Nikolaus [30]	Nutritional risk: well nourished, undernourished	Part of comprehensive geriatric assessment	Physician
Juvenile Rheumatoid Arthritis	Henderson [31]	Dietitian referral: yes, no	During a clinic visit	All health care professionals
Learning Difficulties	Bryan [32]	Nutritional risk: yes, no	Not specified	Carer
Long-term Care Residents	Noel [33]	Send to dietitian, screen in 2 weeks, screen in 4 weeks	On admission and re-screen in 2-4 weeks	Non-professional personnel
Medical and Surgical	Potosnak [34]	Nutritional risk: none, mild, moderate, severe	On admission	Not specified
	Oakley [35]	Dietitian referral for nutritional support: yes, no	On admission and repeat weekly	Nurse
	Elmore [36]	Malnutrition risk: low, high	On admission	Not specified
Oncology	Lundvick [37]	Nutritional risk: yes, no	Within 48 hours of admission	Dietitian
	Latkany [38]	Nutritional risk: low, moderate, high	On admission; re-screen within 7-10 days	Diet technician

Table 3(a). Continued

Population	Lead Author [Reference]	Outcome Variable	Time of Assessment	Intended Administrator
Oral and Maxillo-facial Malignancy	Guo [39]	Nutritional status: well nourished, undernourished, malnourished, severe malnourished	At diagnosis	Not specified
Surgical	Hall [40]	Nutritional status: normally nourished, slightly nourished, moderately undernourished, severely undernourished	After 5 days from admission	Clinical assessor
	Lupo [41]	Nutritional status: normal nourishment, mild, moderate, severe malnutrition	Before surgery	Clinical assessor
	Scanlan [42]	Nutritional risk: minimum, at risk, high, very high	On admission and reassess at least weekly	Nurse
	Thompson [43]	Referral of information to physician to decide whether further nutritional assessment is indicated: yes, no	Within 48 hours of admission and at 2 week intervals	Dietitian
	Baker [44]	Nutritional status: normal, mild, severe malnutrition	Before surgery	Clinical examiner
Trauma	Cooper [45]	Malnutrition risk: minimal, significant, high	Within 24 hours of admission and re-screen at least weekly	Trauma nurse

Table 3(b). Studies that evaluated an existing or modified nutritional tool: Outcome variable, time of assessment and administrator

Population	Lead Author [Reference]	Outcome Variable	Time of Assessment	Intended Administrator
Community	Hickson [46]	Nutrition risk: low, medium, high	On admission; repeat if patient's condition changes	Community nurse
Dialysis	Kalantar-Zadeh [47]	Malnutrition score: risk groups not defined	Not specified	Dietitian, nurse, physician
	Enia [48]	Nutritional status: well nourished, moderate, severe malnutrition	End of dialysis/with empty peritoneum	Not specified
	Visser [49]	Nutritional status: well nourished, mild to moderately, severely malnourished	Not specified	Not specified
Elderly Inpatients	Ek [50]	Nutritional status: well nourished, moderately, severely malnourished	Within 1st week of hospital stay	'Trained observer'
Male outpatients	Prendergast [51]	Nutritional risk: low, high	At scheduled appointment	Not specified
Nursing or residential homes	Wright [52]	Nutritional risk: low, needs monitoring, high	On admission and when cause for concern	Nurse
Gastroenterology	Detsky [53]	Nutritional status: well nourished, moderately or suspected, severely malnourished	Before surgery	Physician, nurse
	Hirsch [54]	Nutritional status: well nourished, moderately, severely undernourished	Within 4 days of admission	To include less experienced professional
HIV Infected	Bowers [55]	Nutritional status: well nourished, mild to moderately, severely malnourished	At out-patients and subsequent follow-up visit	Dietitian, nurse and other health care professional
Liver Transplant	Hasse [56]	Nutritional status: well nourished, moderately or suspected, severely malnourished	As part of liver transplant evaluation	Not specified
Medical and Surgical	Brown [57]	Nutritional risk: none, mild, moderate, severe	On admission; reassess during stay	Nurse

Professional Group(s) of Administrators

There is clearly quite an array of intended users of the tools. Many were developed for just one professional group, such as, nurses or dietitians, whereas others were intended for an assortment of health professionals. A few were developed for relatively untrained and unskilled personnel, and even the patient. For one tool [25], different professional groups were responsible for different sections of the form, which was then evaluated by a medical/dietetic team. However, three [34,36,39] of the 32 original tools and four [48,49,51,56] of the 12 existing or modified tools did not specifically state the intended administrator of the tool.

Review Conclusion

It is clear that the authors of many published tools have not given sufficient attention to the details regarding a tool's application. Without this information being precisely defined, it is impossible for potential users to know whether they are correctly applying the tool. A tool used inappropriately will not provide useful data, resulting in the likely misclassification of nutritional status.

B. Tool Development

Suppose that we have identified a tool suitable for the intended population, which has a clear definition of its application. We now turn our attention to its development. We want to be confident that the tool has been developed using an appropriate method, is based on factors known to be associated with malnutrition, but on the other hand, does not contain unnecessary information. In addition, we need to ensure that the process of obtaining a subject's nutritional state is consistent with the skills of the intended administrator. Moreover, there must be evidence that the tool has been pre-tested to assess its ease of use and acceptability to both its administrators and target population. Finally, of course, it must have been published to allow us the opportunity of using it. Criteria to assess a tool's development are listed in Table 4 and described in further detail below. The appropriate features of each tool identified by the literature search were appraised accordingly.

Table 4. Criteria for assessing a nutritional tool: Development

TOOL DEVELOPMENT
Content
Content based on literature search and experience
Assessment of content validity
Format
Implementation of a pilot study
Presentation of the tool
Derivation
Method used to determine the best predictors of malnutrition
Evidence of scientific rigour in the tool's derivation

Content

The starting point to tool development is the compilation of risk factors that are known or believed to be associated with malnutrition in the intended subject population. These can be obtained from a literature search, existing instruments or clinical experience of malnutrition. For potential users to be confident that the tool comprises important risk factors which are evidence based, it is important to reference the source of each variable. Practical considerations regarding the choice of variables or questions include availability, the time frame for the evaluation, the expertise of the tool's administrators, and the intended subject population.

Content Based on Literature Search and Experience
Twenty two (69%) of the 32 studies that presented an original tool gave some form of justification for the tool's content. An example of referencing selected variables is provided by Ferguson *et al.* [22], but few other papers gave such citations.

Content Validity
Once the risk variables have been assembled, it is important to check the content validity of the collection. This involves an independent judgment of the relevance and completeness of the selection by an expert group but only one [15] of the reviewed tools specifically stated that they assessed content validity.

Format

Proforma Design

Having established that the selection of questions and variables has content validity, the next step is to lay them out as a proforma or questionnaire. Careful thought should be given to the layout of the form, instructions for completion and question sequence [59]. Questions should be formulated so that they are clearly expressed, easily understood and free from the effect of bias [63].

Pilot Study

Before recommending the tool for use, it is essential to perform a pre-test or pilot study, which allows all aspects of the tool usage to be tested. This can identify:

- difficulties in accessing subjects within the clinical setting at the appropriate times at which the tool should be used
- problems with obtaining information in the tool
- that the tool can be administered within a realistic time frame
- training needs of users and the format that this should take
- problems with the content and layout of the tool.

Appropriate modifications to the tool and its usage can also be made based on the users' comments, suggestions and criticisms. Typically, a pilot study may involve forty subjects and several users (eight to ten say), with each user administrating the tool to four or five subjects [59].

Only five studies identified by the literature review reported a pilot of their new tool to determine ease of use and completeness. Following use of their tool, six studies assessed its acceptability and identified the need for further modifications to the form, the production of a training package, or instruction manuals to minimise misunderstandings amongst users. Based on feedback from users, three studies that applied a modified version of a tool concluded that further changes were needed.

Presentation of Tool

Most studies used a proforma or questionnaire to determine nutritional status or risk of malnutrition but two developers of original tools did not publish this [16,27].

Derivation

Redundant Variables Excluded

Although we require a tool to be based on the important risk factors associated with malnutrition, we do not want it to include redundant information. It is likely that there will be some overlap in the initial choice of risk variables, and we may find that we have two or more variables measuring a similar facet of nutritional risk. How do we decide whether just one of these variables is sufficient to represent this aspect of risk, and which should we use? An important feature of tool development should be the sifting of the original set of risk factors to determine those which are the best predictors of malnutrition, and hence base the tool on the smallest number of relevant variables.

All but four studies took their initial choice of variables to be the nutritional screening or assessment tool. The following four tools were derived following a reduction of their initial selection of variables to arrive at a subset which was highly associated with malnutrition. One study [36] used discriminant analysis to identify the best indicators of malnutrition, and another [17] used both discriminant and multiple regression analyses. The other two studies [22,31] used trial and error to arrive at a combination of variables with the highest sensitivity and specificity when compared with a gold standard. Ferguson *et al.* [22] chose the subjective global assessment [53] as the gold standard for defining malnutrition, Elmore *et al.* [36] used a full nutrition assessment, and the other two studies [17,31] used dietitians assessment of available information.

The method for obtaining nutritional status or risk for each tool was identified and classified into four approaches:

- subjective assessment of data i.e. without the use of a pre-defined algorithm
- use of pre-defined criteria or questions
- sum of scores applied to the responses of pre-defined variables
- other analytical procedure

The decision to use a subjective or analytical approach to obtain nutritional state may be due to personal preference but may also depend upon the situation in which the tool will be applied. A subjective approach allows an observer to make a clinical judgement based on available data, perhaps in association with guidelines, but may be less effective when used by less experienced or trained personnel.

Tables 5(a) and 5(b), respectively, present the method used by developers of a new tool, and for tools that were either evaluated in a new population or were modifications of an existing tool. All but one study [47] that evaluated an existing or modified tool used a similar method to that of the original tool.

Subjective Assessment

Four (12%) of the 32 original tools and seven (58%) of the 12 studies that evaluated or modified an existing tool obtained nutritional status based on a subjective assessment of data. All seven studies of existing or modified tools were based on a modified version of one of these instruments, namely, the subjective global assessment [44].

Pre-Defined Criteria

Eleven (34%) of the 32 original tools and two (17%) of the 12 studies that evaluated or modified an existing tool obtained nutritional status using a criteria based approach, as described below.

Four studies [20,25,31,32] defined nutritional risk according to whether specific responses were given or criteria met. Clark *et al.* [14] also defined criteria for recommending nutrition referral but these were not given in the paper. They carried out a logistic regression analysis to develop a model for predicting which variables on the screening form were most likely to result in a nutrition referral, and recommended amending their initial criteria to incorporate some of the variables identified by this analysis.

Two studies [26,38] graded the severity of risk for each variable and defined a patient's nutritional risk status by the number and severity of risk factors. Potosnak *et al.* [34] recorded each variable as normal or abnormal and defined the degree of nutritional risk by the number of abnormal criteria; this tool was evaluated by Brown and Stegman [57]. Thompson *et al.* [43] used a similar approach and defined nutritional risk if significant abnormal parameters were identified but this was not quantified. Wolinsky *et al.* [19] used a series of questions having yes/no responses and defined nutritional risk if a certain number of 'yes' responses were obtained; this tool was evaluated by Prendergast *et al.* [51]. Wolinsky *et al.* [19] justified the number of 'yes' responses associated with nutritional risk from analyses that indicated that this was the most powerful for discriminating between at risk and not at risk groups with respect to health status and health services utilisation. Nikolaus *et al.* [30] also used a sequence of yes/no responses, defining nutritional risk if a certain number of 'yes' replies were given but gave no justification for this particular number.

Table 5(a). Studies that presented an original nutritional tool: Method for obtaining nutritional status

Population	Lead Author [Reference]	Subjective[a] Assessment	Criteria[b] Based	Total[c] Score	Other[d]
Children with Special Health Care Needs	Clark [14]		✓		
	Campbell [15]			✓	
Community Patients	Gilford [16]			✓	
	Ward [17]				✓
Elderly Subjects	Guigoz [18]			✓	
	Wolinsky [19]		✓		
Hospital Patients Adult	Kovacevich [20]		✓		
	Goudge [21]			✓	
	Ferguson [22]			✓	
Hospital Patients Adult+Paediatric	Reilly [23]			✓	
	Nagel [24]			✓	
	Hunt [25]		✓		
Hospital Patients Age not stated	Hedberg [26]		✓		
	Lowery [27]				✓
Hospital Patients Elderly	Pattison [28]			✓	
	Cotton [29]			✓	
	Nikolaus [30]		✓		
Juvenile Rheumatoid Arthritis	Henderson [31]		✓		
Learning Difficulties	Bryan [32]		✓		
Long-term Care Residents	Noel [33]			✓	
Medical and Surgical	Potosnak [34]		✓		
	Oakiey [35]			✓	
	Elmore [36]				✓
Oncology	Lundvick [37]	✓			
	Latkany [38]		✓		
Oral and Maxillo-facial Malignancy	Guo [39]				✓
Surgical	Hall [40]	✓			
	Lupo [41]	✓			
	Scanlan [42]			✓	
	Thompson [43]		✓		
	Baker [44]	✓			
Trauma	Cooper [45]			✓	

[a] No pre-defined algorithm
[b] Pre-defined criteria or questions
[c] Sum of scores allocated to responses of pre-defined variables
[d] Other analytical procedure

Table 5(b). Studies that evaluated an existing or modified nutritional tool: Method for obtaining nutritional status

Population	Lead Author [Reference]	Subjective[a] Assessment	Criteria[b] Based	Total[c] Score	Other[d]
Community	Hickson [46]			✓	
Dialysis	Kalantar-Zadeh [47]			✓	
	Enia [48]	✓			
	Visser [49]	✓			
Elderly Inpatients	Ek [50]	✓			
Male outpatients	Prendergast [51]		✓		
Nursing or residential homes	Wright [52]				✓
Gastroenterology	Detsky [53]	✓			
	Hirsch [54]	✓			
HIV Infected	Bowers [55]	✓			
Liver Transplant	Hasse [56]	✓			
Medical and Surgical	Brown [57]			✓	

[a] No pre-defined algorithm
[b] Pre-defined criteria or questions
[c] Sum of scores allocated to responses of pre-defined variables
[d] Other analytical procedure

Total Score

An analytical approach used by thirteen (41%) of the 32 original tools and by three (25%) of the 12 studies that evaluated or modified an existing tool was to obtain nutritional status by firstly allocating a numerical score to each category of the variables thought to be related to malnutrition. Similarly, numerical variables were grouped and given a score. The score for each variable was summed and the total score was then assumed to represent the risk of malnutrition. Risk groups of malnutrition were defined by categorising the total score. Three studies [16,23,47] did not clarify how the risk groups could be obtained from the total score.

The scores applied to each risk category should reflect that variable's effect on malnutrition. Hence scientific reasoning should be provided for their magnitude and for the range of the total score corresponding to risk of malnutrition. Only a few of the studies attempted to justify this. Campbell and Kelsey [15] based the score on a variable's relative nutritional importance, and used clinical judgement to define the range. Cotton *et al.*

[29] based both the scores and range of the total score associated with malnutrition on clinical judgement. Goudge *et al.* [21] allocated a 'relevant' score, whereas Reilly and colleagues [23] designed their scoring system to reflect the risk of under-nutrition. Oakley and Hill [35] devised their weighting by reviewing existing scoring systems, discussions within the dietetic department and using existing patient records. Ferguson and her colleagues [22] chose the scoring system to give the highest sensitivity and specificity when compared to a gold standard of Subjective Global Assessment [53].

Three studies justified the range corresponding to risk of malnutrition using an analytical approach [18,22,35]. Ferguson *et al.* [22] chose the cut-off value with the highest sensitivity and specificity, and Guigoz *et al.* [18] selected the cut-off points as a result of tabulating the score with albumin. An interim analysis led Oakley and Hill [35] to change their cut-off value to increase specificity.

It is problematic to know how each risk variable should be weighted. As this approach pre-judges the effect of a variable on malnutrition, it may be dependent upon the clinical experience of the tool's developers. Although a handful of studies gave a considered approach to choice of scores and ranges corresponding to risk groups of malnutrition, it is difficult not to get the impression that some studies appeared to use an arbitrary system and hence overlooked the importance of this critical aspect of tool development.

Other Analytical Procedure

Four (12%) of the 32 original tools used some other analytical approach to obtain nutritional status. Lowery *et al.* [27] also allocated numerical scores to the responses of variables but used an algorithm of averages, rather than the total score, to obtain nutritional status but did not clearly define in the paper how this could be determined. Guo *et al.* [39] also used an algorithm to compute the general nutritional status score, which was grouped into grades of malnutrition but no justification for these groupings was given.

Two studies obtained nutritional status from the results of multivariate analyses using a multiple regression model [17] or discriminant equation [36]. Results from these analyses were used to weight the risk variables according to the strength of their relationship with malnutrition.

Review Conclusion

It is evident from this review, that there is no uniform procedure for developing a nutritional screening or assessment tool. An apparent lack of scientific rigour in the development of some of the tools casts doubt on their value and usefulness. In particular, the majority of tools based on a total score approach, appeared to use an arbitrary scoring system, and hence overlooked the importance of this critical aspect of tool development. This led the author to previously conclude that use of a multivariate procedure, based on well established principles of design and analysis, could significantly increase advancement of research into the identification of factors associated with malnutrition [13].

There is no doubt that multivariate models have been developed and used successfully in many areas of medicine [64-66] and by different professional groups, and the author strongly believes that they could play an important role in the development of nutritional screening and assessment tools. Practical aspects of achieving this using a multivariate technique have been published [59]. However, the fact that only two tools were developed using a multivariate procedure may suggest that researchers are unfamiliar with such an approach or are unaware of its potential benefits. The following section gives an outline of the method for using a particular multivariate analysis (linear logistic regression) to derive a tool, comparing and contrasting it with the other analytical procedures previously used for nutritional tool development. Practical suggestions are made regarding the formation of an appropriate dataset. The merits and usefulness of this multivariate technique for tool development are highlighted. The dissent to multivariate procedures from a few authors of nutritional tools is considered.

Chapter 3

MULTIVARIATE ANALYSIS

First, let us consider some of the advantages. A multivariate analysis will:

- determine whether all the initially chosen risk variables are needed to predict malnutrition
- identify a subset of the best indicators of malnutrition
- weight these important risk factors according to their effect on malnutrition
- generate a formula for estimating the probability of malnutrition for a given subject as a function of these risk factors
- use the formula to assign a subject to a group reflecting his or her estimated malnutrition risk, such as, at risk, not at risk.

Hence the analysis will help ensure that the tool does not contain superfluous information, will derive scores (or weights) for the risk variables, and incorporates a procedure for combining these scores to obtain an overall risk of malnutrition, which can then be used as a risk classification rule. It clearly overcomes the arbitrariness and lack of scientific rigour which characterises the development of some of the tools previously described in this book.

Dataset

Design issues considered in the earlier sections of this book relating to tool application, content, and format, apply regardless of the method used to develop a tool. However, a major difference between the previously described methods of using pre-defined criteria or sum of scores to obtain nutritional status and the usage of a multivariate technique is the creation of an appropriate dataset. The multivariate approach requires data to be collected from subjects in the population for which the tool is intended.

A detailed account of how this dataset should be formed is given in Jones [59]. Subjects should be selected using random or convenience sampling, recruited as a single cohort unclassified by nutritional state and from a clinical setting and point in the referral process where the tool would be used, with the selection and referral processes fully described [67]. For each subject, we record data on the potential risk factors and also require an assessment of a subject's 'true' nutritional status from a gold standard procedure. It is important to ensure that the same information is collected for each subject because missing data may introduce bias into the dataset. This can occur if the missing data do not occur at random but are associated with malnutrition, thereby influencing the identification of the important risk factors.

The gold standard procedure should be detailed with positive and negative diagnoses clearly defined [67]. It should be available for all subjects, based on the same tests and/or information in all subjects, with blinding procedures to ensure all assessments are independent. Ideally the gold standard is an accepted, clearly defined and documented, objective evaluation for diagnosing malnutrition. However, the absence of such a standard gives rise to a number of problems. In particular, a subjective assessment of data arising from a gold standard procedure with unknown reliability is likely to require repeat assessments. This will be considered later under the section on Criterion Validity.

As discussed previously, the risk groups associated with the tool's outcome variable should be defined in association with distinct action plans. However, using a multivariate technique, the number of categories used by the gold standard is another factor to consider when determining the risk groups for the tool. The ideal option is to link the categories of the tool with those of the gold standard. For example, suppose that the gold standard procedure allocates subjects to one of two groups (such as, undernourished or adequately nourished). If the tool also allocates subjects to two groups (such as, at risk, no risk), then a cross-tabulation of these two variables allows an evaluation of the tool's performance in relation to the gold standard. However, if the tool allocates subjects to more than two groups (such as, at risk, probable risk, no risk), it is unclear how to handle the middle group(s) when comparing the tool's performance with the gold standard [59]. The assumption will now be made that both the gold standard and the tool allocate a subject to one of two groups, such as, undernourished/adequately nourished for the gold standard and at nutritional risk/not at risk for the tool.

Another aspect that must be addressed is the number of subjects we need to recruit into the study. This is dependent upon the estimated prevalence of malnutrition in the target population and the number of variables to be included in the multivariate analysis. Prevalence of malnutrition may be estimated by looking at research carried out in a similar population, or obtained from a pilot study. Jones [59] suggests the following approach for sample size determination. Suppose we wish to develop a tool for a population in which M% are expected to be malnourished, and let p represent the number of variables to be included in the multivariate analysis. For the tool to give good discrimination between groups of malnourished and nourished subjects, the minimum sample size is 1000p/M if M does not exceed 50%, or 1000p/(100-M) if M is greater than 50% [68], with the proviso that at least 100 subjects are recruited.

For example, suppose we wish to develop a tool for adult acute in-patients, with an estimated prevalence of malnutrition of 40%, based on 25 dichotomous risk variables. The minimum sample size for a multivariate analysis is thus 1000x25/40 = 625 subjects. A study using 25 dichotomous risk factors amongst people with disabilities, of whom 55% are expected to be at nutritional risk would require data collecting on 1000x25/(100-55) = 556 subjects.

Prior to analysis, extensive checking of the dataset is vital to remove all inaccuracies and inconsistencies.

Univariate Analysis

A univariate analysis is an essential first step prior to a multivariate analysis. Standard methods of analysis (described in [59]) are used to compare the characteristics of subjects identified by the gold standard as being undernourished with those of subjects deemed to be adequately nourished. This allows a careful examination of the nature of a possible relationship between a risk variable and malnutrition, and hence suggests the optimal way(s) to handle the variable in the subsequent multivariate analysis, as illustrated below.

Data from a study [17] that developed a tool for assessing risk of under-nutrition in patients in the community were reanalysed by Jones [59]. Of particular note is the effect of body mass index (BMI) on malnutrition rates. Studies that have included BMI as a risk factor in their nutritional tool, tend to assume that the higher the BMI, the lower the risk of malnutrition; that is, a linear relationship. However, a consideration of malnutrition rates by groupings of BMI showed that rates initially decreased with increasing BMI but then increased for values of BMI greater than 28 (Table 6). This suggested a quadratic rather than a linear effect of BMI on malnutrition. Unlike the pre-defined criteria and sum of scores methods, it is not necessary to group a numerical variable for inclusion in a multivariate method. The actual value of BMI was used in this analysis, and a quadratic function of BMI proved to be the most significant variable associated with undernutrition.

Table 6. Effect of body mass index on risk of malnutrition [59] using data from a published study [17]

Variable	Level	Number of subjects: At risk/Total	At risk of malnutrition (%)
Body mass index (kg/m^2)	<18	27/30	90.0
	18-19.9	30/44	68.2
	20-21.9	36/51	70.6
	22-23.9	31/65	47.7
	24-25.9	25/78	32.1
	26-27.9	17/77	22.1
	28-29.9	14/49	28.6
	30+	30/112	26.8

Univariate analysis of a categorical variable compares the malnutrition rates between the different categories. If this reveals a small number of subjects in some of the groups, it would be sensible to combine these with other categories of the variable if this makes sense from a nutritional or clinical perspective and if the malnutrition rates in these groupings appear similar. If the cross-tabulation reveals that no subject had a particular characteristic of nutritional risk, this zero count will cause difficulties in the subsequent model fitting process. Options to deal with this include combining categories of the variable in a meaningful way or eliminating the category completely.

The univariate analysis can only assess the importance of each risk factor by itself. However, some variables may only appear to be significant because they are correlated with other variables that are in fact significant. In order to identify those variables that are independently related to malnutrition, the relative importance of the variables can be examined simultaneously using a multivariate technique.

Multivariate Analysis

The linear logistic regression analysis is a powerful multivariate technique for analysing data in which the response variable can have only one of two possible values (such as, undernourished or adequately nourished). The associated formula, termed a model, is of the form:

$$\log_e [p/(1-p)] = \beta_0 + \beta_1 X_1 + \beta_2 X_2 + \ldots + \beta_k X_k$$

where p is the probability of malnutrition, the X's denote the risk variables and the β's are associated parameters or weights. The weights are estimated from the data using a method called maximum likelihood. A full description of the linear logistic regression model is given by Hosmer and Lemeshow [69]. Several statistical programs carry out this analysis, such as SPSS [70] and Minitab [71].

The model is often derived using a stepwise procedure in which variables are selected either for inclusion or exclusion from the model in a sequential fashion. Forward selection with a test for backward elimination is a stepwise process commonly employed. This involves defining two p values, one for selecting variables for entry into the model (p_E) and the other for removing variables from the model (p_R). To derive a tool comprising a small number of variables, p_E could be set to 0.05, and to avoid removing many variables once they have entered, p_R could be set to 0.9. A likelihood ratio chi-square test is used to assess the significance of a variable. The end result of the analysis is identification of a subset of risk variables related to malnutrition, and estimation of their associated weights.

Jones [59] illustrates this methodology using data from a published nutritional study [17]. The multivariate analysis reduced the initial set of 26 risk factors (age, BMI and 24 dichotomous questions) to a subset of four variables. The weights given to these variables are given in Table 7, together with the model formula for combining these scores to give the probability of malnutrition for a subject, and an example of its usage.

Table 7. Results of a multivariate analysis [59] of data from a published study [17]

Variable	Variable Name	Maximum Likelihood Estimate of Regression Coefficient	Standard Error of Estimate
Constant		9.134	1.691
Body mass index	BMI	-0.664	0.117
Body mass index squared	BMISQ	0.010	0.002
Clothing recently feels loose	V1=0 if no =1 if yes	0.960	0.222
Often feels full very quickly	V2=0 if no =1 if yes	0.937	0.234
Needs help with cooking	V3=0 if no =1 if yes	0.691	0.216

Model Formula
Probability of malnutrition = $\dfrac{e^S}{1 + e^S}$

where $S = 9.134 - 0.664\,(BMI) + 0.01\,(BMI^2) + 0.96\,(V1) + 0.937\,(V2) + 0.691\,(V3)$

Example
Patient with BMI=20.5, clothing has not recently felt loose (V1=0), often feels full very quickly when starting to eat (V2=1) and needs help with cooking (V3=1)

$S = 9.134 - 0.664 \times 20.5 + 0.01 \times 20.5^2 + 0.96 \times 0 + 0.937 \times 1 + 0.691 \times 1 = 1.3525$

Probability of malnutrition = $e^{1.3525} / (1 + e^{1.3525})$
= 0.795

Nutritional Screening Tool

The factors, which are identified by the multivariate analysis as being the best indicators of malnutrition, form the nutritional screening tool. Before adopting this as the method for assessing nutritional risk, it is advisable to first pilot it, as described previously under the 'Format' section of tool development.

The model formula estimates the probability of malnutrition and is used to classify a subject into a nutritional risk group (such as, at risk or not at risk). This is achieved by using a cut-off value, predicting risk of malnourishment for subjects whose probability exceeds the cut-off and not at risk if the probability is less than the cut-off point. The effectiveness of the allocation rule can be assessed by considering a number of measures, such as, sensitivity (proportion of undernourished subjects identified by the tool as at risk) and specificity (proportion of adequately nourished subjects identified by the tool as not at risk). As these two values may vary substantially according to the cut-off point, a receiver operating characteristic (ROC) plot of sensitivity against (1-specificity) is useful for identifying a cut-off value that produces acceptable levels of sensitivity and specificity, as illustrated in Jones [59]. This must be determined with regard to the consequences of misclassification, with the correct classification of subjects who are malnourished taking precedence over misclassifying adequately nourished subjects [20,22].

An alternative to having a paper based nutritional screening tool is to use one linked to a computer database, which comprises details of the subjects, their medical care and nutritional support. It would be a relatively simple matter to program the model formula (like the example in Table 7) and formation of the resultant nutritional risk groups into the database. Input of the relevant nutritional risk details on admission and at other time-points as specified in the tool's protocol of usage, would generate a patient's nutritional status and make the user aware of the necessary action plan. A history of the patient's nutritional state would thus be routinely preserved in the database. Help options to assist users to collate the relevant information for the risk factors, such as, definitions, measurement particulars and explanatory notes, and the generation of reminders to carers to obtain the required support or to repeat screening could be incorporated into the process.

Evaluation

Various summary measures are computed to estimate a tool's performance. For example, the area under a ROC curve gives a measure of the model's ability to discriminate between those at risk of malnutrition and those not at risk. The area ranges from zero to one, with a value between 0.7 and 0.8 suggesting acceptable discrimination, 0.8 to 0.9 excellent, and greater than 0.9 outstanding discrimination [69].

A comparison of the model's predicted outcomes with the observed outcomes is termed 'goodness of fit'. A number of statistical tests, such as the Hosmer-Lemeshow test [69], assess the overall goodness of fit of the logistic regression model. The Hosmer-Lemeshow test computes the probability of malnutrition for each subject, ranks the probabilities, and then groups them into ten categories of approximately equal size, which are tabulated against a subject's 'true' nutritional status. The goodness of fit statistic is obtained by comparing the observed number of subjects in each category with the number that would be expected under the assumption that the model fits the data.

An evaluation of a tool's performance will produce overly optimistic results if the same data are used both to derive the model and to evaluate its performance. The ultimate aim of evaluating the model formula is to establish that it works satisfactorily for patients other than those from whose data it was derived. Model validation therefore involves use of data from a new set of subjects at the study centre to verify that the tool is suitable for all such people rather than being specific to the characteristics of those in the original dataset. Furthermore, an assessment of whether the tool is transportable to other centres requires an evaluation on data collected from an appropriate subject population at a different centre.

Finally, we need evidence that the tool is both valid and reliable. A detailed discussion of these two concepts is given later in the book.

Modifications

Once a tool has been derived, it is important to regularly monitor its performance. An ongoing collection of data provides opportunities to periodically update the instrument. A tool may need to change with time due to a number of reasons. For example, further research may suggest new risk variables to be included in the analysis, and this may result in a different tool with a better performance than the original. It is also to be expected that the inevitable changes to the general pattern of life, and in the provision of medical care, that take place over a period of time will have an effect on the ability of a tool to accurately identify subjects at risk [72]. This would then require either an update of the existing instrument or the derivation of a new one.

Other Multivariate Techniques

This book has concentrated on just one particular multivariate procedure, namely the linear logistic regression analysis, because it is felt that this is the most appropriate for nutritional tool development. However, a limitation of this method is that the gold standard procedure for obtaining a subject's 'true' nutritional status can have only two possible outcomes, such as, undernourished or adequately nourished.

Elmore *et al.* [36] used discriminant analysis to identify the best indicators of malnutrition, taking the gold standard to be a full nutrition assessment which classified a patient as being either at high risk of malnutrition or at low risk. An advantage of the discriminant is that it can also be used with a gold standard comprising more than two possible outcomes. The relative merits of the linear logistic regression and discriminant analyses have been studied by many researchers, and the general consensus is that the performance of the logistic regression method is superior when analysing risk variables that are categorical or have non-normal distributions [73]. Hence the linear logistic method is likely to be more relevant than the discriminant since many of the potential risk factors related to malnutrition are categorical.

Ward *et al.* [17] used multiple regression analysis to select the predictors of under-nutrition, taking dietitians' diagnosis (four risk groups) as the gold standard. However, this assumption that risk group can be considered a numerical variable is questionable and hence multiple regression analysis is not recommended.

Factor analysis is an item-reducing technique widely used in the development of an instrument for describing a trait or behaviour, which is impossible to measure explicitly. As part of the process, it is required to show that the items have face validity (they appear to measure what they are supposed to measure) and internal consistency (they measure different aspects of the same trait). By considering the correlations between items, factor analysis reduces the number of items. However, the method is not recommended with dichotomous items because the correlations are highly unreliable [74]. Moreover, Streiner and Norman [75] make the important point that these techniques make sense when the aim is to describe a trait but not when the aim is to discriminate people who have an attribute from those who do not. Hence, measures of internal consistency, such as, Cronbach's alpha [76] and factor analysis are unlikely to be appropriate in the development of a nutritional tool to distinguish between different malnutrition risk groups [59].

Further Issues

Multivariate analyses have been criticised by the following developers of nutritional tools. Lowery and her colleagues [27] chose not to base their algorithm on a regression analysis stating that equal weights work just as well and that there is a lack of understanding regarding the meaning of weights developed from regression analysis. The instigators of the subjective global assessment method [44,53] chose a subjective rather than a multivariate approach, citing problems with multivariate analyses if risk variables are correlated with each other.

It is certainly true that numerical problems can occur when fitting a logistic regression model. These problems are caused by the effect that certain data patterns have on the computation of the parameter estimates (weights). This may be a consequence of collinearity (that is, substantial correlation) between risk variables in the model, or, as discussed earlier, due to a zero count in a category of a variable. An extremely large parameter estimate or standard error is often an indication of these numerical problems. Due to these potential difficulties, inexperienced users of multivariate techniques are strongly urged to consult with a statistician. As is the case with any statistical selection process, it is vital to carefully consider the results at each step of the model fitting process to check that they are consistent with clinical knowledge of malnutrition. In conclusion, multivariate modelling by an experienced person is a powerful process for generating valuable results.

C. Tool Evaluation

This third section of methodological appraisal of a tool relates to its performance. We may have comprehensive instructions regarding a tool's application, confidence in its derivation and composition but we also require evidence of its capability. A tool that does not work well may be little more than worthless pieces of paper, the completion of which wastes time and resources. However, its erroneousness in identifying subjects at risk of malnutrition could have serious consequences to patient care. Hence, developers of a tool have an ethical responsibility to provide evidence of its ability.

Performance of an instrument is assessed in terms of reliability and validity. As the methodology and concepts behind both these expressions are different, they will be considered separately.

Chapter 4

RELIABILITY

Reliability measures the agreement between the results of the tool when administered by different users (inter-rater) or on different occasions (intra-rater). Good agreement when more than one user applies the tool to the same subject, at a similar point in time, implies that usage of the tool is not dependent upon the particular user. This assessment of inter-rater reliability should be achievable within most clinical settings. Note that reliability tends to use the term 'rater' to describe the user of an instrument. Intra-rater reliability measures agreement between assessments made on a subject by the same rater or user on two different occasions. This requires the time interval between the two assessments to be chosen such that a subject's nutritional status is unlikely to have changed, but not be too short to introduce memory recall bias. This may be achievable for subjects in long-term care but may be difficult for acute care where length of stay is short and nutritional status may be influenced by intermediary interventions.

This book concentrates on inter-rater reliability as this has the most relevance for nutritional screening and assessment tools. Moreover, demonstration of high inter-rater reliability is sufficient indication of a reliable tool [75].

A reliability study of a new tool should initially be carried out at the centre at which the tool was developed. Publication of these results allows potential users at other centres to decide on the tool's suitability for their particular purpose, and to make comparisons with competing instruments [77]. A high level of reliability may encourage other centres to adopt this tool. However, it cannot be automatically assumed that the tool will work equally well at another centre. Therefore, if a new centre is interested in using the tool, it too must carry out a reliability study to determine how well the tool performs at its site.

The original literature review [13] found that only 20 (45%) of the 44 studies evaluated their tool's reliability, suggesting that researchers are unaware of the importance of measuring reliability. The methodology of each of these twenty reliability studies was appraised. Jones [78] gives a detailed account of the important information, usually incorporated into the study protocol, which should be considered when designing and implementing a reliability study. However, the published accounts of the reliability studies generally gave insufficient information to allow such a comprehensive evaluation. Hence criteria to assess the scientific merit of these studies are limited to those outlined in Table 8. These include design issues, such as, use of intended administrators of the tool, assessment of the independence of ratings, and an appropriate number of raters and subjects. Analysis considerations require the calculation of a relevant measure of reliability. Reliability was considered by thirteen (41%) of the 32 studies that presented an original tool and by seven (58%) of the 12 studies that either evaluated an existing tool in a new population or modified an existing instrument. Information relating to these is presented in Tables 9(a) and 9(b), respectively.

Table 8. Criteria for assessing a nutritional tool: Reliability

TOOL RELIABILITY
Use of intended administrators
Independent assessments by raters
Number of raters specified
Sample size determination for number of subjects
Calculation of a relevant measure of reliability with 95% confidence interval

Two groups of people are required for a reliability study, namely, subjects and raters.

Subjects

As a reliability study should be carried out in the setting in which the tool will be used, subjects must be a representative sample of the target population. They should be selected using random or convenience sampling, with recruitment into the study independent of a subject's nutritional status.

Table 9(a). Studies that presented an original nutritional tool: Reliability

Population	Lead Author [Reference]	Number of Subjects	Number of Raters	Professional Group of Raters	Appropriate Raters	Independent[a] Assessments	Analysis
Community Patients	Gilford [16]	27	2	Community nurses	Yes	Yes	Kappa statistic, Spearman's correlation
Hospital Patients Adult	Kovacevich [20]	186	2	Nurse versus nutritionist	No	Yes	Chi-square goodness of fit test
	Goudge [21]	70	5	Nurses	Yes	Yes	Intra-class correlation
	Ferguson [22]	32	2/3	Dietitians, nutrition assistant	Subset	Yes	Kappa statistic
Hospital Patients Adult+Paediatric	Reilly [23]	20	2	Dietitians	No	Not stated	Spearman's correlation
		19	2	Dietitian versus nurse	No	Not stated	Spearman's correlation
Hospital Patients Age not stated	Lowery [27]	20	54	Dietitians	Yes	Yes	Kappa statistic
			59	Dietetic technicians	Yes	Yes	Kappa statistic
Hospital Patients Elderly	Pattison [28]	66	2	Nurse versus dietitian	Yes	Yes	Weighted kappa statistic
	Cotton [29]	200	2	Nurse versus dietitian	No	Not stated	Wilcoxon matched pair test
	Nikolaus [30]	20	3	Not specified	Not known	Not stated	Pearson's correlation
Learning Difficulties	Bryan [32]	35	3	Nurses	Yes	Yes	Intra-class correlation
Surgical	Hall [40]	46	3	Surgeons	Yes	Yes	Weighted kappa statistic
	Lupo [41]	64	3	Surgeons	Yes	Yes	Kappa statistic
	Baker [44]	59	2	Physicians	Yes	Yes	Kappa statistic

[a] Raters independently used the tool

Table 9(b). Studies that evaluated an existing or modified nutritional tool: Reliability

Population	Lead Author [Reference]	Number of Subjects	Raters	Professional Group of Raters	Appropriate Raters	Independent [a] Assessments	Analysis
Dialysis	Kalantar-Zadeh [47]	12	2	Dietitian versus physician	Subset	Not stated	Kappa statistic
	Visser [49]	22	2	Nurses	Not known	Not stated	Intra-class correlation
Elderly Inpatients	Ek [50]	90	2	Clinician versus researcher	Yes	Yes	Kappa statistic
Male outpatients	Prendergast [51]	41	Not stated	Not stated	Not known	Not stated	Correlation
Gastroenterology	Detsky [53]	109	2	Nurse versus physician	Yes	Yes	Kappa statistic
	Hirsch [54]	175	2	1st year resident versus clinical nutrition specialist	Yes	Yes	Kappa statistic, correlation
Liver Transplant	Hasse [56]	20	2	Dietitians	Not known	Yes	Kappa statistic

[a] Raters independently used the tool

Raters

Each rater independently administers the nutritional tool to each subject. As a reliability study should be implemented in accordance with the tool's intended usage, raters must be chosen from the professional group(s) who will be administering it. This assessment of the reviewed publications is hampered by the fact that full particulars of a tool's usage were often not reported, as observed previously in the Tool Application section.

All thirteen studies that presented the reliability of a new tool, defined their intended administrator and all but one [30] identified the study administrator or rater. Four [47,50,53,54] of the seven studies that evaluated the reliability of an existing or modified tool defined both the intended administrators and raters, two studies [49,56] defined only the raters, and the remaining study [51] gave no indication of either the intended users or the raters.

The reliability of three tools developed for nurses were also assessed by dietitians [20,23,29]. However, use of raters who are not the intended administrators of the tool will yield no information regarding the tool's reliability in its planned setting. Nine (69%) of the thirteen studies of a new tool and four (57%) of the seven studies that evaluated or modified an existing tool were thus identified as using appropriate administrators.

Because tool usage may depend upon a user's expertise or training [28,50], it has been suggested that reliability is assessed separately for each group of intended users [78]. This approach was taken by Lowery *et al.* [27]. However, Ferguson *et al.* [22] used only a subset of the types of people who will be using their tool, and Kalantar-Zadeh *et al.* [47] used raters from only two of their three professional groups of intended administrators.

Independent Assessments

To obtain an unbiased estimate of reliability, all raters must work independently of one another. All but six studies stressed this important feature.

Sample Size

The number of subjects in the reviewed studies ranged from 12 to 200. One study [51] did not state how many raters were used. All but two of the remaining studies used two or three raters.

Although sample size is an essential feature of any investigation, only three studies considered how this should be determined. Kovacevich *et al.* [20] computed the number of subjects, Bryan *et al.* [32] considered both the number of subjects and raters, and Lowery *et al.* [27] having determined the number of subjects by time restraints, calculated the number of raters.

Sample size calculation allows the tool to be evaluated on an adequate number of subjects to give a high probability of estimating its reliability to within a chosen accuracy. Too small a sample will lead to a wide confidence interval, making it difficult to draw conclusions regarding the tool's reliability. It has been argued that such a study will be of little scientific value and hence unethical in its use of subjects, whereas too large a sample will waste resources and impinge unnecessarily on the time of all those involved [78].

The number of subjects required depends on the number of raters. As the number of raters assessing each subject increases, the number of subjects required decreases. The greatest saving in sample size occurs when the number of raters increases from two to three, a gain which gradually diminishes and becomes negligible beyond five raters [79]. There is thus little point in designing a reliability study with more than five raters, and it is likely that the choice would be between two or three raters.

Jones [78] considered the practical implications of using two versus three raters. A possible disadvantage of using two raters is that more subjects are required. However, as most tools are developed for use in a large population, recruitment of enough subjects will not usually be an issue. It may, however, be more problematic for a tool developed for a specialized population, for which use of three raters would clearly be advantageous. Unfortunately, a major obstacle is that the standard error of the kappa statistic (considered in the following 'Methodology' section) for more than two raters is difficult to calculate, and hence confidence intervals and sample size determination are not readily available. It was therefore suggested that reliabilÙ(y studies of nutritional tools are designed using two raters, and this number is assumed in this book. A multi-centre approach to estimating a tool's reliability for a relatively small specialized population would increase the number of available subjects.

Perhaps it is not surprising that so few reliability studies considered sample size, as this is a complex issue. Not only are there several ways to approach the topic depending on the statistical assumptions made and consequently more than one formula may exist for a given problem, but the resultant formulae are complex, do not usually allow calculation by hand, and are not generally incorporated into computer packages. In view of this, Jones [78] presented a relatively simple approach for the estimation of sample size for a reliability study of a nutritional tool. An extension of this work is presented in the following 'Methodology' section.

Analysis

Nine (69%) of the thirteen studies that presented the reliability of a new tool and six (86%) of the seven studies that evaluated or modified an existing tool analysed their data using a measure of agreement, namely, the kappa statistic or intra-class correlation. (Deliberation on these measures of agreement is given in the 'Methodology' section). The remaining five studies that performed an incorrect analysis used a measure of association [23,30,51], a test of averages [29], or a goodness of fit test [20].

REVIEW CONCLUSION

The review of published nutritional tools thus revealed that less than half the studies evaluated reliability. Of those that did, some gave inadequate attention to important design issues, such as, independent assessments and use of appropriate administrators, a quarter used an incorrect method of analysis and very few considered sample size. To help ensure that future reliability studies of nutritional tools are designed with sufficient numbers of subjects and analysed using appropriate methods, the relevant methodology is dealt with in the following section.

METHODOLOGY FOR RELIABILITY STUDY

The outcome variable associated with a nutritional tool usually has two categories (dichotomous data), or more than two risk categories that are ordered (ordinal data). Since sample size and method of analysis depend on the type of outcome variable, these will be considered separately. A discussion will also be given about the appropriateness of basing an assessment of reliability on a numerical measure of nutritional risk.

Dichotomous Data

Dichotomous data arise when the outcome variable associated with the nutritional instrument has two categories, such as, at nutritional risk or not at risk.

A typical layout of the data resulting from a reliability study is presented in Table 10. Each rater has independently used the tool to make a nutritional assessment of each subject. We wish to estimate the tool's reliability by measuring the level of agreement between the assessments of the two raters.

Both raters gave an assessment of at-risk to five subjects but we can see that these are not always given to the same subject. We have a total of six agreements: three subjects for whom the raters agreed that the patient is at nutritional risk, and three subjects for whom the raters agreed that the patient is not at risk. But the raters disagreed for four subjects: subjects 1 and 7 were assessed to be at nutritional risk by rater 2 but not by rater 1, whereas subjects 8 and 9 were assessed to be at nutritional risk by rater 1 but not by rater 2.

Table 10. Typical layout of data from a reliability study: Agreement between two raters on assessment of nutritional risk

Subject	Rater 1	Rater 2	Agreement
	Subject at nutritional risk		
1	No	Yes	No
2	No	No	Yes
3	No	No	Yes
4	Yes	Yes	Yes
5	No	No	Yes
6	Yes	Yes	Yes
7	No	Yes	No
8	Yes	No	No
9	Yes	No	No
10	Yes	Yes	Yes
Number of 'yes'	5	5	
Number (%) of agreements			6 (60%)

Cross-tabulation of the assessments of one rater with those of the other (Table 11), clearly shows what we have already observed that the raters agreed for six subjects but not for the remaining four. A simple measure of agreement is to calculate the proportion or percentage of subjects for which both raters agreed. The raters agreed for six of the ten subjects, giving an agreement rate of 60%. However, this measure does not allow for the possibility that some of the agreement will be due to chance. For example, if the raters had determined nutritional risk randomly using the toss of a coin (with say, a 'tail' indicating at-risk and a 'head' not at-risk), then there would still be some agreement between them. So, when measuring agreement, it is essential to report the agreement that is observed over and above that which would be expected simply due to chance. Such a statistic is the kappa statistic [80] – a chance corrected index of agreement, usually denoted by κ.

Table 11. Cross-tabulation of the risk assessments of ten subjects by two raters

At Nutritional Risk?		Rater 2		Total
		Yes	No	
Rater 1	Yes	3	2	5
	No	2	3	5
Total		5	5	10

Table 12 gives a general layout of results and formulae for the calculation of a kappa statistic for two raters and dichotomous data; these are now used to analyse the data in Table 11. The observed agreement has already been calculated as 60%, so the observed proportion $p_0 = 0.6$. The agreement expected by chance, $p_e = (5 \times 5 + 5 \times 5)/10^2 = 0.5$.

Hence kappa = $\dfrac{0.6 - 0.5}{1 - 0.5}$ = 0.2

The formulae for kappa and its standard error are in terms of observed agreement (denoted by p_0) and expected agreement (p_e), as follows:

$$\text{Kappa} = \frac{p_0 - p_e}{1 - p_e}$$

Standard error of kappa (SE) = $\sqrt{\dfrac{p_0(1-p_0)}{N(1-p_e)^2}}$

where the observed agreement is the proportion of subjects for which raters agree, that is,

$p_0 = (a+d)/N$, and the expected agreement $p_e = (R_1 \times C_1 + R_2 \times C_2)/N^2$

The 95% confidence interval for kappa is given by the formula:

kappa ± 1.96 x SE

Table 12. Calculation of the kappa statistic for two raters, dichotomous outcome variable

At Nutritional Risk?		Rater 2		Total
		Yes	No	
Rater 1	Yes	a	b	R_1=a+b
	No	c	d	R_2=c+d
Total		C_1=a+c	C_2=b+d	N

We would now like to know whether this indicates that the tool has adequate reliability. This is a difficult question to answer precisely because there are no objective criteria by which to judge kappa. It is known that kappa has a value of zero when agreement is no better than chance and a maximum of 1.0 when agreement is perfect. To interpret values within this range, Landis and Koch [81] proposed the classification scheme shown in Table 13. This was discussed by Shrout [82] who argued for a stricter classification, which has the effect of moving the labels up one category (Table 13). The author shares the view that the descriptions given by Landis and Koch are too generous, and hence recommends that reliability is interpreted using Shrout's scheme. Hence a kappa of 0.2 indicates only slight agreement over and above what we would expect due to chance.

In practice, it is more informative to report the value of kappa with a confidence interval. Several formulae exist for the standard error of kappa and hence the confidence interval. A relatively simple formula is presented in Table 12, although it has the disadvantage of overestimating the standard error and hence gives a conservative confidence interval [83]. Although the adjective label of agreement is usually chosen to describe the estimated value of kappa, it can also be applied to the confidence interval. If the reliability study has been performed with a small number of subjects, it is likely that the confidence interval covers a range of labels, indicating that the study has provided little useful information regarding the tool's reliability. An example of the calculation and interpretation of a confidence interval for kappa is given in Jones [78].

Table 13. Two schemes for the interpretation of reliability

Landis and Koch [81]		Shrout [82]	
Value of reliability	Strength of agreement	Value of reliability	Strength of agreement
<0.00	Poor		
0.00-0.20	Slight	0.00-0.10	Virtually none
0.21-0.40	Fair	0.11-0.40	Slight
0.41-0.60	Moderate	0.41-0.60	Fair
0.61-0.80	Substantial	0.61-0.80	Moderate
0.81-1.00	Almost perfect	0.81-1.00	Substantial

Clearly, the above example is based on an unrealistically small number of subjects. Suppose we wish to design a reliability study in which enough subjects are recruited to be 95% confident that the value of kappa obtained from the sample will be within a certain distance of the true value of kappa. The required sample size for a reliability study with a dichotomous outcome variable depends upon:

- An estimate of kappa in the study population. The ability to estimate reliability to within a certain degree of accuracy depends upon its actual value. For a study of an existing tool, the estimate of reliability reported by the tool's developers can be used. For a new tool, implementation of a pilot study will enable estimation of kappa.
- An estimate of the prevalence of malnutrition in the study population. This can be obtained by looking at research carried out in a similar population.
- The level of the confidence interval for kappa. This book considers only a 95% confidence interval because it tends to be standard practice to calculate this interval for a statistic.
- The level of precision to which it is required to estimate kappa; this is termed the maximum error. The smaller this value, the greater the precision and the larger the required number of subjects. How do

we decide upon an appropriate value? The 95% confidence interval for kappa is of the form κ±d, where d is the maximum error. A suitable value for d must be determined based upon the range of values that kappa can take (usually between 0 and 1) and in the context of the groupings used to describe the strength of agreement. As adjectives used to describe reliability (Table 13) mostly correspond to intervals of 0.2, it has been suggested [78] that an appropriate value for the maximum error is 0.1 since this results in a 95% confidence interval of width 0.2. This value will be assumed in this book.

Several approaches exist for determining sample size [84-86]. Because the adequacy of these methods depend on the use of large sample estimates of the standard error of kappa and on the approximate normality of the distribution of kappa, caution should be exercised if a sample size of less than 100 is indicated [86]. Hence figures presented in this paper are based on a minimum sample size of 100. Table 14 presents sample size figures based on Cantor's method [84], which has the advantage that it allows sample size to be estimated in circumstances where raters differ in their proportions of at-risk subjects. Sample size for a confidence level other than 95% and a maximum error of kappa other than 0.1 can be obtained from Cantor's paper [84].

Determination of sample size will be illustrated using hypothetical data from a pilot reliability study (Table 15), which will be used to calculate the sample size for the main study. It can be seen from Table 15 that rater 1 assessed 14 out of 45 subjects as at-risk (31%) and rater 2 assessed 10 out of 45 (22%). These two percentages will be rounded to 30% and 20% respectively. The value of kappa was calculated to be 0.663 implying moderate reliability (Table 13). From Table 14, the sample size for 30% and 20% at risk and a kappa of 0.6 is 311, and for a kappa of 0.7 is 249. Taking the larger of these two values gives an estimated sample size for the reliability study of 311 subjects.

The rounding of the at-risk percentages and reliability value is a limitation of the usage of Table 14. For investigators with access to SPSS, Figure 2 presents SPSS commands which allow a more accurate determination of sample size. This requires the user to input values of the four figures a, b, c, and d, as defined in Table 12 into SPSS variables named A, B, C and D respectively. The SPSS routine can either be run by entering and running each line one by one in the Transform → IF and/or Compute option, or by entering all the commands in a SPSS syntax window and running them in one go. The required sample size figure is variable *SSIZE*. Output using this routine on the data in Table 15 gives a sample size figure of 266 (Figure 3). A reliability study of 266 subjects would thus allow the researchers to be 95% confident that the value of kappa obtained from their study would be within 0.1 of the true value of kappa.

Table 14. Sample size for a reliability study assuming dichotomous outcome variable, two raters, 95% confidence interval for kappa and maximum error of 0.1

Percentage at risk		Estimate of kappa					
Rater 1	Rater 2	0.4	0.5	0.6	0.7	0.8	0.9
10	10	848	801	705	569	401	209
20	10	548	512	448			
20	20	489	451	392	314	222	116
30	10	350					
30	20	394	360	311	249		
30	30	379	344	296	236	167	100
40	20	297	268				
40	30	334	300	257	205		
40	40	335	301	257	205	145	100
50	20	207					
50	30	272	243	207			
50	50	323	289	246	196	139	100
60	30	202					
60	40	264	235	200			
60	50	310	277	237	189	133	
60	60	335	301	257	205	145	100
70	40	202					
70	50	272	243	207			
70	60	334	300	257	205		
70	70	379	344	296	236	167	100
80	50	207					
80	60	297	268				
80	70	394	360	311	249		
80	80	489	451	392	314	222	116
90	70	350					
90	80	548	512	448			
90	90	848	801	705	569	401	209

COMPUTE ROW1 = A + B.
COMPUTE ROW2 = C + D.
COMPUTE COL1 = A + C.
COMPUTE COL2 = B + D.
COMPUTE TOTAL = A + B + C + D.
COMPUTE A11 = A / TOTAL.
COMPUTE A12 = B / TOTAL.
COMPUTE A21 = C / TOTAL.
COMPUTE A22 = D / TOTAL.
COMPUTE B11 = ROW1 * COL1 / TOTAL**2.
COMPUTE B12 = ROW1 * COL2 / TOTAL**2.
COMPUTE B21 = ROW2 * COL1 / TOTAL**2.
COMPUTE B22 = ROW2 * COL2 / TOTAL**2.
COMPUTE P0 = A11 + A22.
COMPUTE PE = B11 + B22.
COMPUTE KAPPA = (P0 - PE) / (1.0 - PE).
COMPUTE C11 = (ROW1 + COL1) / TOTAL.
COMPUTE C22 = (ROW2 + COL2) / TOTAL.
COMPUTE C12 = (ROW2 + COL1) / TOTAL.
COMPUTE C21 = (ROW1 + COL2) / TOTAL.
COMPUTE D11 = ((1.0 - PE) - (1.0 - P0) * C11)**2.
COMPUTE D22 = ((1.0 - PE) - (1.0 - P0) * C22)**2.
COMPUTE NUM1 = A11 * D11 + A22 * D22.
COMPUTE NUM2 = (A12*(C12**2) + A21*(C21**2)) * (1.0 - P0)**2.
COMPUTE NUM3 = (P0 * PE - 2 * PE + P0)**2.
COMPUTE Q = (NUM1 + NUM2 - NUM3) / (1.0 - PE)**4.
COMPUTE SIZE = 1.0 + Q / (0.1/1.96)**2.
COMPUTE SSIZE = TRUNC(SIZE).
IF (SSIZE LT 100) SSIZE = 100.
EXECUTE.

Note
1. The SPSS commands are not case sensitive.
2. Spaces in the formulae on the right hand side of '=' are not necessary.
3. Variable S†'ZE gives the required sample size, and variable KAPPA gives the value of kappa. Values of all other intermediary variables can be deleted from the resultant database.
4. The 'Execute' command is not required, if each line is entered and run one by one in the Transform → Compute or IF option

Figure 2. SPSS routine to calculate the sample size for a reliability study assuming the tool has two risk categories, two raters, 95% confidence interval for kappa and maximum error of 0.1

Case Summaries

A	B	C	D	KAPPA	SSIZE
9	5	1	30	.6625	266

Figure 3. Output from SPSS routine (Figure 2) to calculate the sample size for a reliability study (assuming tool has two risk categories, two raters, 95% confidence interval for kappa and maximum error of 0.1) applied to data in Table 15

Table 15. Hypothetical data from a pilot reliability study with a dichotomous outcome variable

At Nutritional Risk?		Rater 2		Total
		Yes	No	
Rater 1	Yes	9	5	14
	No	1	30	31
Total		10	35	45

Observed agreement, $p_0 = (9 + 30) / 45 = 0.8667$

Expected agreement, $p_e = (14 \times 10 + 31 \times 35) / 45^2 = 0.6049$

$$\text{Kappa} = \frac{0.8667 - 0.6049}{1 - 0.6049} = 0.663$$

Ordinal Data

Ordinal data occur when the response variable associated with the nutritional tool has ordered categories. Examples include nutritional risk classified as none, mild, moderate or severe, and nutritional status ordered as well nourished, moderately malnourished or severely malnourished.

The calculation of kappa can be extended fairly easily to agreements with more than two categories. An example of the calculation is given in Table 16 using hypothetical data from a pilot reliability study. An example of the calculation and interpretation of a confidence interval for kappa for ordinal data is given in Jones [78].

Table 16. Hypothetical data from a pilot reliability study with an outcome variable having three categories

Nutritional Risk		Rater 2			Total
		Low	Moderate	High	
Rater 1	Low	13	3	2	18
	Moderate	4	13	2	19
	High	1	2	20	23
Total		18	18	24	60

Observed agreement (p_0) is the proportion of subjects for which raters agree:

$p_0 = (13 + 13 + 20) / 60 = 0.7667$

Using similar notation to Table 12,

$$\text{expected agreement, } p_e = (R_1 \times C_1 + R_2 \times C_2 + R_3 \times C_3) / N^2$$
$$= (18 \times 18 + 19 \times 18 + 23 \times 24) / 60^2$$
$$= 1218 / 3600 = 0.3383$$

$$\text{Kappa} = \frac{p_0 - p_e}{1 - p_e} = \frac{0.7667 - 0.3383}{1 - 0.3383} = 0.647$$

An alternative analysis of ordinal data is to compute a weighted kappa, in which the disagreements are weighted according to the number of groups separating the assessments of the two raters. Two of the reviewed studies [28,40] computed this statistic but did not define the weights.

It has been suggested [78], based on the following reasons, that the unweighted kappa is preferable. Firstly, there is no general agreement regarding the choice of weights, with differing schemes being recommended [87,88]. Secondly, as reliability depends upon the choice of weights, it is difficult to compare the reliability of tools for which different weighting systems have been used. Thirdly, it is difficult to choose weights that reflect the relative seriousness of disagreement between users on a subject's clinical management. If a weighted kappa is used, the weighting system should be justified, and both weighted and unweighted kappas presented.

COMPUTE ROW1 = V11 + V12 + V13.
COMPUTE ROW2 = V21 + V22 + V23.
COMPUTE ROW3 = V31 + V32 + V33.
COMPUTE COL1 = V11 + V21 + V31.
COMPUTE COL2 = V12 + V22 + V32.
COMPUTE COL3 = V13 + V23 + V33.
COMPUTE TOTAL = ROW1 + ROW2 + ROW3.
COMPUTE A11 = V11 / TOTAL.
COMPUTE A12 = V12 / TOTAL.
COMPUTE A13 = V13 / TOTAL.
COMPUTE A21 = V21 / TOTAL.
COMPUTE A22 = V22 / TOTAL.
COMPUTE A23 = V23 / TOTAL.
COMPUTE A31 = V31 / TOTAL.
COMPUTE A32 = V32 / TOTAL.
COMPUTE A33 = V33 / TOTAL.
COMPUTE B11 = ROW1 * COL1 / TOTAL**2.
COMPUTE B12 = ROW1 * COL2 / TOTAL**2.
COMPUTE B13 = ROW1 * COL3 / TOTAL**2.
COMPUTE B21 = ROW2 * COL1 / TOTAL**2.
COMPUTE B22 = ROW2 * COL2 / TOTAL**2.
COMPUTE B23 = ROW2 * COL3 / TOTAL**2.
COMPUTE B31 = ROW3 * COL1 / TOTAL**2.
COMPUTE B32 = ROW3 * COL2 / TOTAL**2.
COMPUTE B33 = ROW3 * COL3 / TOTAL**2.
COMPUTE P0 = A11 + A22 + A33.
COMPUTE PE = B11 + B22 + B33.
COMPUTE KAPPA = (P0 - PE) / (1.0 - PE).
COMPUTE C11 = (ROW1 + COL1) / TOTAL.
COMPUTE C22 = (ROW2 + COL2) / TOTAL.
COMPUTE C33 = (ROW3 + COL3) / TOTAL.
COMPUTE C12 = (ROW2 + COL1) / TOTAL.
COMPUTE C21 = (ROW1 + COL2) / TOTAL.
COMPUTE C13 = (ROW3 + COL1) / TOTAL.
COMPUTE C23 = (ROW3 + COL2) / TOTAL.
COMPUTE C31 = (ROW1 + COL3) / TOTAL.
COMPUTE C32 = (ROW2 + COL3) / TOTAL.

Figure 4 continued on next page

COMPUTE D11 = ((1.0 - PE) - (1.0 - P0) * C11)**2.
COMPUTE D22 = ((1.0 - PE) - (1.0 - P0) * C22)**2.
COMPUTE D33 = ((1.0 - PE) - (1.0 - P0) * C33)**2.
COMPUTE NUM1 = A11 * D11 + A22 * D22 + A33 * D33.
COMPUTE NUM2 = (A12*(C12**2)+A21*(C21**2)+A13*(C13**2)+ A23*(C23**2)+ A31*(C31**2)+A32*(C32**2)) * (1.0 - P0)**2.
COMPUTE NUM3 = (P0 * PE - 2 * PE + P0)**2.
COMPUTE Q = (NUM1 + NUM2 - NUM3) / (1.0 - PE)**4.
COMPUTE SIZE = 1.0 + Q / (0.1/1.96)**2.
COMPUTE SSIZE = TRUNC(SIZE).
IF (SSIZE LT 100) SSIZE = 100.
EXECUTE.

Note
1. The SPSS commands are not case sensitive.
2. Spaces in the formulae on the right hand side of '=' are not necessary.
3. Variable SSIZE gives the required sample size, and variable KAPPA gives the value of kappa. Values of all other intermediary variables can be deleted from the resultant database.
4. The 'Execute' command is not required, if each line is entered and run one by one in the Transform → Compute or IF option

Figure 4. SPSS routine to calculate the sample size for a reliability study assuming the tool has three risk categories, two raters, 95% confidence interval for kappa and maximum error of 0.1

As discussed previously, sample size depends on an estimate of kappa in the study population, the coefficient of the confidence interval and the maximum error. Determination of sample size for ordinal data also depends upon the number of response categories, and the percentages of subjects expected in each category. When the frequencies of the categories are approximately equal, the sample size will be smaller than when one or two of the categories are much more frequently used by the raters than the remaining categories [86].

Due to the increased number of factors that influence sample size, it is difficult to include figures for all such possibilities in tabular form. However, sample size for a response variable having three categories can be obtained using the SPSS routine presented in Figure 4. This computes the sample size using the large sample standard error of kappa given by Fleiss et al. [83]. The algorithm requires the user to input values of the nine frequencies from the reliability table in a similar fashion to that for the routine for dichotomous data. The three frequencies for the first row are placed into variables *V11*, *V12* and *V13* respectively, frequencies for the second row into variables *V21*, *V22* and *V23* respectively, those for the third row into variables *V31*, *V32* and *V33* respectively. The SPSS routine can either be run by entering and running each line one by one in the Transform → IF and/or Compute option, or by entering all the commands in a SPSS syntax window and running them in one go. The required sample size figure is variable *SSIZE*.

Determination of sample size will be illustrated using hypothetical data from the pilot reliability study (Table 16), which will be used to calculate the sample size for the main study. Values of the 9 variables *V11* to *V33*, as defined above, are shown in Figure 5. Output using the SPSS routine on this data gives a sample size figure of 154 (Figure 5). A reliability study of 154 subjects would thus allow the researchers to be 95% confident that the value of kappa obtained from their study would be within 0.1 of the true value of kappa.

Case Summaries

V11	V12	V13	V21	V22	V23	V31	V32	V33	KAPPA	SSIZE
13	3	2	4	13	2	1	2	20	.6474	154

Figure 5. Output from SPSS routine (Figure 4) to calculate the sample size for a reliability study (assuming tool has three risk categories, two raters, 95% confidence interval for kappa and maximum error of 0.1) applied to data in Table 16

The SPSS routine in Figure 4 can be fairly easily extended to calculate a sample size for a tool with more than three risk categories, or alternatively assistance may be sought from the author.

Numerical Data

As observed in the Tool Development section, several nutritional tools have been developed using the sum of scores approach, in which the total score is taken to represent a subject's risk of malnutrition. Agreement between total scores may be measured using an intra-class correlation coefficient. This measurement of chance corrected agreement applicable for numerical data is computed by analysing the data using an analysis of variance, which splits the total variability in the data into variability due to different sources. Details and examples have been published [89,90]. Interpretation of reliability can be made using the schemes in Table 13.

However, in practice, nutritional risk is not based on the actual value of the total score but rather on a classification scheme. As was described in the section on Tool Development, the total score is split into two or more predefined risk categories, and a subject's nutritional status is determined according to the category in which the score lies. It is essential that the reliability of a tool is assessed in the setting in which clinical decisions are made. So, although it may be of interest to report the agreement between scores using the intra-class correlation coefficient, the tool's reliability must be based on the analysis of dichotomous or ordinal data using the techniques previously described.

Establishment of Reliability

Having carried out the (inter-rater) reliability study with a sufficient number of subjects, we need to consider the implications of the results. We want to know whether the tool shows adequate reliability to warrant its implementation. Although Shrout [82] states that substantial reliability is the only category where the adjective conveys the sense that measures are generally adequate, it would not be unreasonable to require the tool to have at least moderate reliability. Unfortunately, the majority of reliability studies of a nutritional tool have been implemented with too few subjects to gauge whether an estimated value of kappa and its confidence interval of greater than 0.6 are realistic in this context. Even for a tool that shows such a level of reliability, it would be advisable to repeat the reliability study at regular intervals, perhaps yearly, to remain confident that the tool continues to perform well.

What should we do if the estimated value of kappa and its confidence interval is not particularly high (i.e. reliability is less than 0.6)? Streiner and Norman [75] suggest that an intra-rater reliability study be implemented to see whether this is due to differences within or between raters. However, as previously discussed this may not be workable in an acute care setting.

Inadequate reliability clearly indicates a lack of uniformity in the manner that users apply the instrument. Developers of a new tool need to identify whether this may be due to ambiguity in the wording of questions, with users or subjects interpreting statements differently, or due to non constant measurement techniques. Identification of such problem areas will require refinement of the tool and modifications to training or explanatory notes, followed by a pilot study of its implementation. A reliability study of the modified tool will indicate whether such changes have increased the tool's performance to an acceptable level.

Users of an existing tool should check that the tool is being implemented in strict accordance with the tool's intended usage. Increased reliability may require a more rigorous training programme than that proposed by the tool's developers.

Chapter 5

VALIDITY

Although there may be good agreement between the results of the tool when administered by different users, we need to be confident that the outcome variable is indeed a measure of nutritional risk. Validity indicates whether an instrument measures what it purports to do.

There are a number of ways to approach an assessment of a tool's validity. In the Tool Development section, we saw that content validity was an important evaluation by a group of experts regarding the relevance and completeness of the selection of risk variables on which the tool was to be derived. Other aspects of validity which will now be considered relate to the developed tool.

Construct validity focuses on the extent to which a measure performs in accordance with theoretical expectations [91]. That is, we would expect risk categories of a nutritional tool to differ with respect to variables not used to construct the tool but known to be associated with malnutrition, and not to differ by variables considered independent of malnutrition. If performance of the tool is consistent with these expectations, then construct validity is demonstrated with respect to these variables.

Criterion validity involves a comparison of the tool's assessment of nutritional status with some other measure of nutritional state, ideally obtained using a gold standard procedure. If the tool performs well, good agreement is expected between the two assessments, as indicated by a high level of criterion validity.

It has been noted that one of the most confusing aspects of validity is the terminology, with various terms used to describe the many approaches to assess validity [75,92]. Traditionally, criterion validity has been divided into two types: concurrent and predictive validity. Concurrent validity is a comparison of the tool with a criterion measured at a similar time to the tool, whereas predictive validity compares the tool with a future criterion. More recently, there has been a tendency to use the term predictive validity for a comparison of the tool with any future variable, construct or criterion, and this more obvious meaning has been used in this book. Hence, it will be assumed that assessment of construct and criterion validity relate to quantities measured at a similar time to the tool, whereas, a comparison of the tool with variables, not available until some time in the future, has been termed predictive validity.

A validity study of a new tool should initially be carried out at the centre at which the tool was developed. Publication of these results allows potential users at other centres to decide on the tool's suitability for their particular purpose, and to make comparisons with competing instruments. A high level of validity may encourage other centres to adopt this tool. However, it cannot be automatically assumed that the tool will work equally well at another centre. Therefore, if a new centre is interested in using the tool, it too must carry out a validity study to determine how well the tool performs at its site.

Evaluation of a tool's validity is an on-going process. Several studies may be required to look at construct validity in relation to different parameters, which may generate new hypotheses requiring new studies [75]. Similarly, several studies may be needed to evaluate criterion validity in relation to different gold standards. In addition, use of the tool in a different population requires new validity studies, as does any modification of the tool [75].

As the level of a tool's reliability influences its validity, it is usual to implement a reliability study prior to a validity study. Reliability places an upper limit on validity, such that the higher the reliability, the higher the maximum possible validity [75]. Before implementing a validity study, it would therefore be sensible to introduce measures (such as those discussed at the end of the Reliability section) in order to optimise the tool's reliability.

The original literature review [13] found that approximately two-thirds of the 44 studies evaluated some aspect of their tool's validity, suggesting that some researchers are unaware of the importance of assessing validity. This book presents a more extensive evaluation of the methodology of each of the validity studies than it was possible to include in the original review.

Jones [93] gives a detailed account of the important information, usually incorporated into the study protocol, which should be considered when designing and implementing a validity study. However, the published accounts of the validity studies generally gave insufficient information to allow such a comprehensive evaluation. Hence criteria to assess the scientific merit of these studies are limited to those outlined in Table 17.

Table 17. Criteria for assessing a nutritional tool: Validity

TOOL VALIDITY
Tool Usage
Use of intended administrators
Multiple raters if required
Independent assessments by raters
Blinded to the gold standard, constructs or additional investigations
Method for obtaining a summary measure from multiple raters
Construct Validity
Definitions of constructs
Assessments independent of tool's outcome
Sample size determination for number of subjects
Appropriate method of analysis
Criterion Validity
Procedure for obtaining a subject's 'true' nutritional status
Assessments independent of tool's outcome
Sample size determination for number of subjects
Appropriate method of analysis

These criteria include design issues, such as, use of intended administrators of the tool, assurance that all assessments are independent and the study is implemented with a sufficient number of subjects. Analysis considerations require use of an appropriate statistical technique to analyse validity. Validity was considered by eighteen (56%) of the 32 studies that presented an original tool and by nine (75%) of the 12 studies that either evaluated an existing tool in a new population or modified an existing instrument.

Design issues common to construct and criterion validity are considered in the following section. Because the two types of validity invoke different sample size and methods of analysis, these will be considered separately.

TOOL USAGE

Information relating to application of the tool is presented in Tables 18(a) and 18(b), respectively, for each new tool, and for each existing or modified tool that had validity assessed.
Two groups of people are required for a validity study, namely, subjects and raters.

Subjects

As a validity study should be carried out in the setting in which the tool will be used, subjects must be a representative sample of the target population, selected using random or convenience sampling, with recruitment into the study independent of a subject's nutritional status.

Raters

As a validity study should be implemented in accordance with the tool's intended usage, the study administrators or raters must be chosen from the professional group(s) who will be administering it. This assessment of the reviewed studies is hampered by the fact that full particulars of a tool's usage were often not reported, as observed previously in the Tool Application section.

All but two [36,39] of the eighteen studies that considered the validity of a new tool, defined the intended administrator, and all but five [18,22,30,36,39] identified the study administrator or rater. Three [48,49,51] of the nine studies that evaluated the validity of an existing or modified tool did not define the intended administrator, and three [48,51,57] gave no indication of the study administrator.

Table 18(a). Studies that presented an original nutritional tool: Details of tool application for assessing validity

Population	Lead Author [Reference]	Number of Raters	Professional Group of Raters	Appropriate Raters	Method to Derive a Single Rating	Independent [a] Assessments
Children with Special Health Care Needs	Campbell [15]	1	Primary caregiver	Yes	-	-
Community Patients	Gilford [16]	2	Community nurses	Yes	Analysed separately	Yes
Elderly Subjects	Guigoz [18]	1 assumed	Not stated	Not known	-	-
Hospital Patients Adult	Kovacevich [20]	1	Nurse	Yes	-	-
	Goudge [21]	1 assumed	Nurse	Yes	-	-
	Ferguson [22]	1 assumed	Not stated	Not known	-	-
Hospital Patients Adult+Paediatric	Reilly [23]	2	Dietitians	No	Pooled data	Not stated
	Hunt [25]	1	Multi-disciplinary team	Yes	-	-
Hospital Patients Age not stated	Lowery [27]	54	Dietitians	Yes	Average agreement	Yes
		59	Dietetic technicians	Yes	Average agreement	Yes
Hospital Patients Elderly	Pattison [28]	2	Nurse and dietitian	Yes	Analysed separately	Yes
	Nikolaus [30]	1 assumed	Not stated	Not known	-	-
Learning Difficulties	Bryan [32]	3	Nurses	Yes	Majority opinion	Yes
Medical and Surgical	Oakley [35]	1	Dietitian	No	-	-
	Elmore [36]	1 assumed	Not stated	Not known	-	-
Oral and Maxillofacial Malignancy	Guo [39]	1 assumed	Not stated	Not known	-	-
Surgical	Hall [40]	3	Surgeons	Yes	Analysed separately	Yes
	Lupo [41]	3	Surgeons	Yes	Not stated	Yes
	Baker [44]	2	Physicians	Yes	Unanimous opinion	Yes

[a] Raters independently used the tool

Table 18(b). Studies that evaluated an existing or modified nutritional tool: Details of tool application for assessing validity

Population	Lead Author [Reference]	Number of Raters	Professional Group of Raters	Appropriate Raters	Method to Derive a Single Rating	Independent[a] Assessments
Dialysis	Kalantar-Zadeh [47]	1	Dietitian	Subset	-	-
	Enia [48]	1	Not stated	Not known	-	-
	Visser [49]	2	Nurses	Not known	Not stated	Not stated
Elderly Inpatients	Ek [50]	2	Clinician and researcher	Yes	Analysed separately	Yes
Male outpatients	Prendergast [51]	1 assumed	Not stated	Not known	-	-
Nursing or residential homes	Wright [52]	1	Nurse	Yes	-	-
Gastroenterology	Hirsch [54]	2	1st year resident and clinical nutrition specialist	Yes	Unanimous opinion	Yes
HIV Infected	Bowers [55]	1	Dietitian	Subset	-	-
Medical and Surgical	Brown [57]	1	Not stated	Not known	-	-

[a] Raters independently used the tool

Two developers of a tool intended for nurses, assessed validity using dietitians [23,35]. However, use of administrators who are not the intended users of the tool will yield no information regarding the tool's validity in its planned setting. Eleven (61%) of the eighteen studies of a new tool and five (56%) of the nine studies that evaluated or modified an existing tool were thus identified as using appropriate administrators.

As tool usage may depend upon a user's expertise or training, it has been suggested that validity is assessed for each group of intended users [93]. This was the approach taken by three studies [27,28,50], but two investigations [47,55] used only a subset of the types of people who would be using the tool.

Another factor to consider when designing a validity study is the number of raters that should apply the tool to each subject. If the tool's reliability can be described as at least moderate, then it may be sufficient to depend upon a single rating. Ten of the eighteen studies of a new tool and six of the nine studies that evaluated or modified an existing tool either specifically stated that one rater administered the tool to each subject or, in the absence of any other information, this was assumed. However, some of these did not carry out a reliability study, and hence would not know whether the tool's reliability was high enough to depend upon a single rating.

If there is some doubt regarding the adequacy of the tool's reliability, then it may be advisable for more than one rater to apply the tool to each subject. Eleven studies utilised multiple raters, but the reason for their use is more likely to be an effect of having the same subjects in both the reliability and validity studies. Various methods were used to analyse the resultant multiple assessments for each subject. Four studies [16,28,40,50] evaluated the tool's validity by analysing the data for each rater separately, two studies either averaged or inappropriately pooled the data, and two [41,49] did not indicate their approach. The remaining three studies obtained a single rating for a subject using a majority rule [32] or an unanimity rule [44,54].

Majority and unanimity rules are illustrated in Jones [93] for two and three raters, assuming the tool's outcome can have only two possible values, such as, at risk or not at risk. Both rules are quick and easy to apply, but a disadvantage of the unanimity rule is that a single summary measure cannot be obtained for cases of disagreement. Since these would be excluded from the validity analysis, this approach is wasteful of data. Use of three raters will always allow a majority opinion for two risk categories, but may not give a unique majority for more than two categories. An alternative approach would be to resolve differences by discussion. This may give a more accurate assessment than use of a rule and can be used with any number of raters or risk categories. However, this method is likely to be more time consuming than the majority rule, and may be difficult to co-ordinate if a large number of different raters is involved.

Independent Assessments

To obtain an unbiased estimate of validity, all raters must work independently of one another. All but two studies [23,49] who used multiple raters stressed this important feature.

REVIEW CONCLUSION

It would appear that some studies have not given sufficient attention to detail regarding the design and implementation of the validity study. Such a study is unlikely to provide an unbiased assessment of the tool's validity.

CONSTRUCT VALIDITY

Eight (25%) of the 32 studies of a new tool and seven (58%) of the 12 studies that either evaluated an existing tool in a new population or modified an existing instrument considered construct validity. The choice of constructs, assessment of the independence of these measurements and the tool's outcome, number of subjects and method of analysis are presented in Tables 19(a) and 19(b), respectively, for each new tool, and for each existing or modified tool that had construct validity assessed.

Constructs

Construct validity requires specification of the expected relationships between the tool's outcome with variables not used to construct the tool [93]. Studies assessed construct validity by comparing numerical variables, such as, anthropometric measurements, body mass index and laboratory investigations, between the risk categories of the tool, with the underlying assumption that these would differ by nutritional risk. Such measurements were made at a similar time to usage of the tool.

Table 19(a). Studies that presented an original nutritional tool: Construct validity

Population	Lead Author [Reference]	Construct	Independent [a] Assessments	Number of Subjects	Method of Analysis
Elderly Subjects	Guigoz [18]	Comprehensive nutrition assessment	Not stated	155	Discriminant analysis
Hospital Patients Adult	Ferguson [22]	Anthropometric and biochemical measures	Not stated	408	Analysis of variance
Hospital Patients Elderly	Pattison [28]	Physical measurements	No	66	Correlation
	Nikolaus [30]	Anthropometric and biochemical values	Not stated	126	Correlation
Oral and Maxillo-facial Malignancy	Guo [39]	Nutrition laboratory tests	Not stated	127	t test
Surgical	Hall [40]	Objective nutritional assessment	Yes	46	Spearman's correlation
	Lupo [41]	Objective measures	Yes	64	Analysis of variance, correlation
	Baker [44]	Objective nutritional assessment	Yes	48	Analysis of variance, correlation

[a] Blinding of results from tool usage and construct measurements

Table 19(b). Studies that evaluated an existing or modified nutritional tool: Construct validity

Population	Lead Author [Reference]	Construct	Independent[a] Assessments	Number of Subjects	Method of Analysis
Dialysis	Kalantar-Zadeh [47]	Anthropometric and biochemical measures	Yes	41	Correlation
	Enia [48]	Objective measurements	Yes	59	Correlation
	Visser [49]	Objective nutritional parameters	Not stated	22	Correlation
Elderly Inpatients	Ek [50]	Objective nutritional assessment	Not stated	90	Correlation
Male outpatients	Prendergast [51]	Anthropometric and biochemical measures	Not stated	377	Analysis of variance, correlation
Gastroenterology	Hirsch [54]	Anthropometric and biochemical measures	Yes	139	Analysis of variance
HIV Infected	Bowers [55]	Biochemical measures	Not stated	36	Quoted means in the risk groups

[a] Blinding of results from tool usage and construct measurements

Independent Assessments

Only six studies stressed that the investigations and measurements were made independently and without knowledge of the tool's outcome. By using the same person to apply the nutritional screening tool and to take the physical measurements for each subject, one study [28] clearly did not have an independent evaluation.

Sample Size

The number of subjects in the construct validity studies ranged from 22 to 408, but no study justified their choice of sample size.

Analysis

Standard methods of analysis are required to compare the average response of nutrition parameters across the tool's risk groups. For a tool with two risk groups, the choice of analysis is between the 2 sample t-test and the Mann-Whitney test, depending on whether or not the variable under comparison follows an approximate normal distribution. For a tool with more than two categories, the choice is between analysis of variance (for approximately normally distributed data) and the non-parametric Kruskal-Wallis test. Clearly, selection of the correct technique can only be made having first determined whether the variable under consideration follows an approximate normal distribution but none of the reviewed studies reported that they had explored this.

Five studies, that obtained nutrition status using subjective assessment, performed a correlation analysis between nutritional variables and risk group. However, this assumption that risk group can be considered a numerical variable is questionable and hence correlation is not recommended. Five studies correlated nutritional parameters with a score representing a subject's risk of malnutrition. Although this may be of interest, this does not provide an assessment of the validity of the tool in the context in which nutritional risk is classified.

REVIEW CONCLUSION

The review of published nutritional tools thus revealed that only a third of the studies evaluated construct validity, and of those that did, no justification of the sample size was given. Some studies assessed construct validity using an inappropriate analysis, while others gave no reasoning for their choice of a parametric or non-parametric comparison of averages. Clearly, more careful attention needs to be given to use of the most appropriate method of analysis. However, as no study considered sample size, the methodology associated with this will be considered in the following section to help ensure that future studies of construct validity are designed with sufficient numbers of subjects.

Sample Size for Construct Validity Study

Sample size will be considered assuming that the tool has two possible outcomes, such as, at nutritional risk or not at risk, that the nutritional parameter under consideration follows an approximate normal distribution and that its variance is similar in the two risk groups. Sample size determination for more than two risk categories, for variables that are not normally distributed or do not have constant variance is more involved, and it is suggested that expert statistical advice be sought.

Let us suppose we wish to determine whether construct validity can be established with respect to one particular nutritional measure, namely, triceps skinfold thickness (TSF). We would expect the average value of this variable amongst subjects at risk of malnutrition to differ from that for subjects not at risk. We wish to design the construct validity study so that a sufficient number of subjects is recruited to give a high probability of detecting a clinically or nutritionally meaningful difference in TSF between the two risk groups as being statistically significant, should such a difference exist. The required sample size depends upon:

The definition of a clinically or nutritionally meaningful difference. For example, a large difference, of say, 10 mm in the mean TSF of the two risk groups would be considered of clinical significance, whereas, a small difference of say, 0.5 mm would be too small to have any clinical importance. Somewhere between these two extremes, lies a point at which the magnitude of the difference starts to have clinical or nutritional significance; this is termed the minimum clinical difference. Its value is determined by the investigators in the context of the particular construct validity study.

The variation in the measurements. For a numerical variable, this can be measured by the standard deviation, an estimate of which may be available from previous research carried out in a similar population of subjects.

The probability of detecting a nutritionally meaningful difference, should it exist; this is termed the power of a hypothesis test. Conventionally, this is set to 90%.

The probability of incorrectly concluding that the risk groups differ with respect to TSF; this is termed the significance level. Conventionally this is set to 5%.

Assumption of equal or unequal size risk groups. If the prevalence of malnutrition in the study population is expected to be 50%, this would result in equal size risk groups. A different prevalence level would give rise to risk groups of unequal size.

(1) Equal Size Risk Groups

It is assumed that the variable under analysis follows a normal distribution and that its variance (s^2) is similar in the two risk groups. Equal sized risk groups are also assumed, that is, the prevalence of malnutrition is expected to be 50%. The number of subjects in each risk group (n) to give a 90% chance of detecting the minimum clinical difference (d) at the 5% significance level is given by:

$$n = \frac{21.02 \, s^2}{d^2}$$

For example, suppose the tool under evaluation has been developed for use in a population of adult acute in-patients with an expected prevalence of malnutrition of 50%, and we wish to study its construct validity with respect to triceps skinfold thickness. From past research, an estimate of the standard deviation of TSF is taken to be 8.3 mm and the minimum clinical difference is defined as 5 mm. Use of the above formula gives the minimum number of subjects in each risk group to be $(21.02 \times 8.3^2) / 5^2 = 57.9$. This number is rounded up to 58 in each group, giving a total sample size of 116 subjects. Therefore, measurements of triceps skinfold thickness for 116 subjects are required to be 90% confident of detecting a difference of 5 mm or more at the 5% significance level, with an estimated standard deviation of 8.3 mm and prevalence of malnutrition of 50%.

(II) Unequal Sized Risk Groups

There are many situations where the prevalence of malnutrition is not expected to be 50%. An adjustment is now required to take into account the resultant unequal sized groups [94].

Let R denote the ratio between the numbers of subjects in the two groups, and n the sample size using the formula for equal sized groups. The number of subjects to be studied from the at risk group, n_A, is given by the following formula:

$$n_A = \frac{(1 + R) n}{2R}$$

The number of subjects not at risk, $n_B = Rn_A$, to give a total sample size $N = n_A + n_B$.

For example, suppose the tool under evaluation has been developed for use in a population of adult patients in the community with an expected prevalence of malnutrition of 25%, and we wish to study its construct validity with respect to triceps skinfold thickness. Suppose that from past research, an estimate of the standard deviation of TSF is 8.3 mm and the minimum clinical difference is defined as 5 mm. The ratio between at risk and not at risk is 25:75 or 1:3, giving R=3. Use of the above formula gives $n_A = 4 \times 58 / 6 = 38.7$ (rounded up to 39), and $n_B = 3 \times 39 = 117$, giving a total sample size of 156. Therefore, measurements of triceps skinfold thickness for 156 subjects are required to be 90% confident of detecting a difference of 5 mm or more at the 5% significance level, with an estimated standard deviation of 8.3 mm and prevalence of malnutrition of 25%. Further worked examples of sample size determination for a construct validity study are given in Jones [93].

For investigators with access to SPSS, Figure 6 presents SPSS commands which perform the sample size computations as outlined above. This requires the user to input values of the standard deviation, minimum clinical difference and prevalence into SPSS variables named *s*, *d* and *prev* respectively. The SPSS routine can either be run by entering and running each line one by one in the Transform → IF and/or Compute option, or by entering all the commands in a SPSS syntax window and running them in one go. The required sample size figure is variable *SSIZE*. Output using this routine on the two worked examples relating to TSF is given in Figure 7.

COMPUTE NTEMP = TRUNC ((2 * (s * (1.96 + 1.282) / d) **2) + 1).
IF (PREV LT 50) R = (100 - PREV) / PREV.
IF (PREV GE 50) R = PREV / (100 - PREV).
COMPUTE NATMP = (1 + R) * NTEMP / (2 * R).
COMPUTE NA = TRUNC (NATMP + 1).
IF (NA - NATMP = 1) NA = NA - 1.
COMPUTE NBTMP = (R * NA).
COMPUTE NB = TRUNC (NBTMP + 1).
IF (NB - NBTMP = 1) NB = NB - 1.
COMPUTE SSIZE = NA + NB.
EXECUTE.

Note
1. The SPSS commands are not case sensitive.
2. Spaces in the formulae on the right hand s4Œe of '=' are not necessary.
3. Variable SSIZE gives the required sample size. Values of all other intermediary variables can be deleted from the resultant database.
4. The 'Execute' command is not required, if each line is entered and run one by one in the Transform → Compute or IF option

Figure 6. SPSS routine to calculate the sample size for a construct validity study assuming the tool has two risk categories, the nutritional variable under analysis follows an approximate normal distribution with constant variance, power = 90% and significance level = 5%

Case Summaries

S	D	PREV	SSIZE
8.30	5.00	50.00	116
8.30	5.00	25.00	156

Figure 7. Output from SPSS routine (Figure 6) to calculate the sample size for a construct validity study of triceps skinfold thickness, using data from the two examples in the text. It is assumed that the tool has two risk categories, TSF follows an approximate normal distribution with similar variance in the two risk groups, power = 90% and significance level = 5%

Establishment of Construct Validity

As validity is a matter of degree and not an all-or-none property [91], an unqualified statement that construct validity is established should always be avoided. If performance of the tool is consistent with expectations concerning the nutritional parameters, then construct validity is established only in relation to those particular measures. There is always, of course, the possibility that future studies of additional variables may not perform as hypothesized [93]. If a variable does not behave as expected, then either the initial hypothesis is incorrect or the tool is unable to adequately discriminate between risk groups with respect to this variable. Results of validity studies for the tool carried out amongst different subjects, or from validity studies for other nutritional instruments may help to clarify the reason why the tool lacks construct validity for that particular variable.

CRITERION VALIDITY

Twelve (38%) of the 32 studies of a new tool and two (17%) of the 12 studies that either evaluated an existing tool in a new population or modified an existing instrument considered criterion validity. The choice of gold standard, assessment of the independence of these measurements and the tool's outcome, number of subjects and method of analysis are presented in Tables 20(a) and 20(b), respectively, for each new tool, and for each existing or modified tool that had criterion validity assessed.

Gold standard: Criterion validity involves a comparison of the tool's assessment of nutritional status with that obtained using a gold standard. As there is no generally accepted clinical definition of malnutrition and hence no single gold standard for determining nutrition status [61], the procedure for obtaining a patient's 'true' nutritional status, not surprisingly, varied considerably.

Some studies involved nutritional assessment by a dietitian using a standard protocol or questionnaire [15,21,35], or with an existing nutritional screening tool [16,23]. Bryan et al. [32] used the majority opinion of dietitians who were unfamiliar with the nutritional screening tool, whereas Lowery et al. [27] used the consensus of the expert group of dietitians who had researched and developed their system. Four studies [18,30,36,52] used an unstructured nutritional assessment by a physician or dietitian. The remaining three studies [20,28,50] based their gold standard on objective criterion, such as the use of published normal ranges for measurements.

Table 20(a). Studies that presented an original nutritional tool: Criterion validity

Population	Lead Author [Reference]	'Gold Standard' Process	'Gold Standard' Outcome Variable	Independent[a] Assessments	Number of Subjects	Method of Analysis
Children with Special Health Care Needs	Campbell [15]	Nutrition assessment by 2 dietitians using a standard protocol with queries decided by 3rd dietitian	Nutrition related problems: yes, no	Yes	79	Specificity and sensitivity
Community Patients	Gilford [16]	Dietitian's assessment with an edited version of Wolinsky's Nutritional Risk Index [19]	Not clear	Yes	27	Kappa statistic, Spearman's correlation
Elderly Subjects	Guigoz [18]	Nutrition assessment by 2 physicians; not stated how single measure was formed	Normal, malnourished	Yes	155/120	Prinicipal component and discriminant analyses
Hospital Patients Adult	Kovacevich [20]	Pre-albumin levels	Low, normal	Not stated	56	Specificity and sensitivity
	Goudge [21]	Nutrition assessment by dietitian using questionnaire	At risk: yes, no	Not stated	73	Kappa statistic
Hospital Patients Adult+Paediatric	Reilly [23]	Wolinsky's Nutritional Risk Index [19] Dietitian's clinical impression	Risk: low, moderate, high	No No	20	Spearman's correlation Spearman's correlation
Hospital Patients Age not stated	Lowery [27]	Consensus of expert group of dietitians	Not clear	Yes	20	Agreement rate

Table 20(a). Studies that presented an original nutritional tool: Criterion validity (continued)

Population	Lead Author [Reference]	'Gold Standard' Process	'Gold Standard' Outcome Variable	Independent[a] Assessments	Number of Subjects	Method of Analysis
Hospital Patients	Pattison [28]	Physical measurements of nutritional status	Nourished, undernourished	No	66	Agreement rate
Elderly	Nikolaus [30]	Nutrition assessment by physician	Undernourished, well nourished, obese	Yes	126	Correlation, Mann-Whitney test
Learning Difficulties	Bryan [32]	Majority opinion of 3 dietitians' assessments using their own methods	At risk: yes, no	Yes	35	Kappa statistic
Medical and Surgical	Oakley [35]	Nutrition assessment by dietitian using questionnaire	Needs nutrition support: yes, no	No	118	Specificity and sensitivity
	Elmore [36]	Full nutrition assessment	Malnutrition risk: high, low	Not stated	151	Specificity and sensitivity

[a] Blinding of results from tool usage and gold standard measurements

Table 20(b). Studies that evaluated an existing or modified nutritional tool: Criterion validity

Population	Lead Author [Reference]	'Gold Standard' Process	'Gold Standard' Outcome Variable	Independent[a] Assessments	Number of Subjects	Method of Analysis
Elderly Inpatients	Ek [50]	Objective nutritional assessment	Malnourished: yes, no	Not stated	90	Kappa statistic
Elderly in nursing or residential homes	Wright [52]	Dietitian's assessment	At risk, monitor, low risk	Not stated	15	Agreement

[a] Blinding of results from tool usage and gold standard measurements

An important characteristic of criterion validity for a nutritional tool is clearly the subjective evaluation of data arising from the gold standard process. In the analysis of subjective data, we must allow for the possibility that experts may differ in their interpretation of this data, leading to discordance regarding a subject's 'true' nutritional status. Use of a standardized procedure or structured proforma may help to reduce disagreements. However, if no information exists regarding the reliability of the gold standard method, it is recommended [93] that more than one expert applies the procedure to each subject, working independently and unaware of the results of the tool. To minimise any contamination between the tool and gold standard, experts should be chosen who are not familiar with the tool. A summary measure of the gold standard can be obtained using the majority rule or consensus approach, as previously described.

A precise definition of the outcome groups associated with the gold standard was not always presented. Lowery *et al.* [27] probably used the same four categories of nutrition status as that defined for their tool. There was a lack of clarity regarding the two studies [16,23] that used the Nutritional Risk Index [19]. Reilly *et al.* [23] appeared to have three risk categories associated with this tool, although it had originally been defined with two [19]. Six studies used both a tool and gold standard with two outcome groups, and one study [52] had three risk groups for both the tool and gold standard. Three studies [18,28,50] used a tool with three categories and a gold standard with two, and the remaining study [30] used a tool with two categories and a gold standard with three.

Independent Assessments

Only six studies stressed the independence of the tool's outcome and the gold standard procedure. By using the same person to apply the nutritional screening tool and to make the nutritional assessment using the gold standard, three studies [23,28,35] clearly did not have an independent evaluation.

Sample Size

The number of subjects in the criterion validity studies ranged from 15 to 155; only two studies [20,32] considered how this was determined.

Analysis

Cross-tabulation of the tool's evaluation of nutritional status with that of the gold standard illustrates the level of agreement between the two procedures. This is illustrated in Table 21, assuming that both the gold standard and the tool allocate a subject to one of two groups, such as, undernourished or adequately nourished for the gold standard and at nutritional risk or not at risk for the tool. Only one [50] of the five studies that used a tool and gold standard with differing number of categories clearly indicated how categories were combined to allow a comparison of the two sets of outcomes.

A tool's performance is generally summarized by its sensitivity and specificity. Sensitivity is defined as the percentage of undernourished subjects identified by the tool as being at risk, and specificity is the percentage of adequately nourished subjects identified as not at risk. Four studies of a tool and gold standard procedure both having two outcome groups measured criterion validity using specificity and sensitivity. Formulae for confidence intervals are presented in Table 21. These are valid if frequencies a to d exceed ten. An example of the calculation and interpretation of the confidence intervals for specificity and sensitivity is given in Jones [93].

Table 21. Criterion validity: Summary measures from cross-tabulation of the tool's assessment with a gold standard

		Gold Standard		Total
		Undernourished	Adequately Nourished	
Tool's assessment	At risk	a	b	a+b
	Not at risk	c	d	c+d
Total		N_1=a+c	N_2=b+d	N

Sensitivity, $S = 100a / N_1$
Specificity, $P = 100d / N_2$
95% confidence interval for sensitivity is: $S \pm 1.96 \sqrt{\{S(100-S) / N_1\}}$
95% confidence interval for specificity is: $P \pm 1.96 \sqrt{\{P(100-P) / N_2\}}$

Unbiased estimates of sensitivity and specificity will not be obtained if the gold standard procedure is subject to error. The lack of a generally accepted gold standard for determining nutrition status is clearly an impediment for estimating the diagnostic accuracy of a nutritional tool. Under the assumption that the gold standard is an alternative technique to the tool, designed to give a truer reflection of a subject's nutritional status, it could be argued [93] that it may be more prudent to analyse the data using a measure of agreement, such as, the kappa statistic. Four studies measured criterion validity using kappa statistic. Three studies inappropriately quoted agreement rates (not chance corrected), and others used a measure of association.

REVIEW CONCLUSION

The review of published nutritional tools thus revealed that only a third of the studies evaluated criterion validity. Some papers did not give a clear description as to how the categories of the tool were compared with those of the gold standard, and some did not have independent assessments. Not all studies used an appropriate analysis, and very few considered sample size. To help ensure that future studies of criterion validity are designed with sufficient numbers of subjects, the relevant methodology is considered in the following section.

Sample Size for Criterion Validity Study

If, as discussed above, the assumption is made that the gold standard is an alternative technique to the tool, and therefore criterion validity will be measured using a kappa statistic, the methods for sample size determination presented under the Reliability section could be applied to the design of the criterion validity study. Sample size determination for estimation of a tool's performance in relation to specificity and sensitivity is described below.

Suppose we wish to design a criterion validity study in which enough subjects are recruited to be 95% confident that the value of sensitivity (or specificity) obtained from our sample will be within a certain distance from the true value. The required sample size depends upon:

- An estimate of sensitivity (or specificity) in the study population. The ability to estimate these quantities to within a certain degree of accuracy depends upon their actual values. For a study of an existing tool, estimates of sensitivity and specificity reported by the

Validity

- tool's developers can be used. For a new tool, implementation of a pilot study will provide estimates.
- An estimate of the prevalence of malnutrition in the study population. This can be obtained by looking at research carried out in a similar population.
- The level of the confidence interval for sensitivity (or specificity). This book considers only a 95% confidence interval because it tends to be standard practice to calculate this interval for a statistic.
- The level of precision to which it is required to estimate sensitivity (or specificity). This is termed the maximum error of the estimate.

The decision to base sample size on sensitivity or specificity may depend on which of these is considered to be the more important or on the practicalities of recruiting a sufficient number of subjects. The appropriate formulae to allow sample size calculation are presented below. These formulae are valid if all frequencies a to d in Table 21 are expected to be at least ten.

(I) Sensitivity

To design a criterion validity study in which enough subjects are recruited to be 95% confident that the value of sensitivity (S) obtained from our sample will be within a certain distance (E_1) from the true value, the required number of undernourished subjects is given by the formula:

$$N_A = \frac{1.96^2 \, S \, (100-S)}{E_1^2}$$

If M% of subjects are undernourished, then the total sample size equals $100N_A/M$.

(II) Specificity

To design a criterion validity study in which enough subjects are recruited to be 95% confident that the value of specificity (P) obtained from our sample will be within a certain distance (E_2) from the true value, the required number of adequately nourished subjects is given by the formula:

$$N_B = \frac{1.96^2 \, P \, (100-P)}{E_2^2}$$

If M% of subjects are undernourished, then the total sample size equals $100N_B/(100-M)$.

Determination of sample size will be illustrated using data from one of the reviewed papers [20]. It will be assumed that the validity data from this study (Table 22) is from a pilot, which will be used to calculate the sample size for the main study. Suppose that it is desired to recruit enough subjects to be 95% confident that the values of sensitivity and specificity obtained from the study will be within 5 percentage points of their true values. Data from the pilot estimate the prevalence of malnutrition as 23.2%, sensitivity as 84.6% and specificity as 62.8%, which give rise to sample sizes of 867 and 468 respectively (Table 22). If the latter is considered a more achievable sample size, then a validity study of 468 subjects would thus allow the researchers to be 95% confident that the value of specificity obtained from the study would be within 5 percentage points of the true value. Further worked examples of sample size determination for a criterion validity study are given in Jones [93].

Table 22. Criterion validity: Calculation of sample size using data from a published study [20]

		Gold Standard		Total
		Undernourished	Adequately Nourished	
Tool's assessment	At risk	11	16	27
	Not at risk	2	27	29
Total		13	43	56

Sensitivity = 100 x 11 / 13 = 84.6%
Specificity = 100 x 27 / 43 = 62.8%
Prevalence of under-nutrition = 100 x 13 / 56 = 23.2%

(i) Estimate of sensitivity = 84.6%; maximum error of estimate = 5%

$$N_A = \frac{1.96^2 \times 84.6 \,(100-84.6)}{5^2} = 200.2$$

Therefore undernourished subjects = 201.
Total sample size = 100 (201)/23.2 = 866.4, rounded up to 867 subjects.

(ii) Estimate of specificity = 62.8%; maximum error of estimate = 5%

$$N_B = \frac{1.96^2 \times 62.8\,(100-62.8)}{5^2} = 358.98$$

Therefore adequately nourished subjects = 359.
Total sample size = 100 (359)/(100-23.2) = 467.4, rounded up to 468 subjects.

COMPUTE NA = TRUNC ((1.96**2 * SENS * (100 - SENS) / SENSPREC**2)+1).
COMPUTE NATMP = 100 * NA / PREV.
COMPUTE SENSSIZE = TRUNC (NATMP + 1).
IF (SENSSIZE - NATMP = 1) SENSSIZE = SENSSIZE - 1.
COMPUTE NB = TRUNC ((1.96**2 * SPEC * (100 - SPEC) / SPECPREC**2)+1).
COMPUTE NBTMP = 100 * NB / (100 - PREV).
COMPUTE SPECSIZE = TRUNC (NBTMP + 1).
IF (SPECSIZE - NBTMP = 1) SPECSIZE = SPECSIZE - 1.
COMPUTE SSIZE = MIN (SENSSIZE, SPECSIZE).
COMPUTE MALN = RND (PREV * SSIZE / 100).
COMPUTE NOURISH = SSIZE - MALN.
COMPUTE A = RND (SENS * MALN / 100).
COMPUTE C = MALN - A.
COMPUTE D = RND (SPEC * NOURISH / 100).
COMPUTE B = NOURISH - D.
EXECUTE.

Note:
1. The SPSS commands are not case sensitive.
2. Spaces in the formulae on the right hand side of '=' are not necessary.
3. Variable SENSSIZE gives the sample size for sensitivity, and variable SPECSIZE gives the sample size for specificity. Variables A to D give the expected numbers of subjects in the contingency data, based on the smaller of SENSSIZE and SPECSIZE, to allow the user to check that these are greater than 10. Values of all other intermediary variables can be deleted from the resultant database.
4. The 'Execute' command is not required, if each line is entered and run one by one in the Transform → Compute or IF option.

Figure 8. SPSS routine to calculate the sample size for a criterion validity study for a 95% confidence interval for sensitivity (SENS) with a maximum error of estimate (SENSPREC), and for a 95% confidence interval for specificity (SPEC) with a maximum error of estimate (SPECPREC)

(iii) Check numbers are large enough to use these formulae:

Let sample size = 468 subjects
Expected number:
   Malnourished = 23.2% x 468 = 109; Nourished = 468-109=359
   Malnourished and identified at risk, a, = 84.6% x 109 = 92
   Malnourished and identified not at risk, c, = 109-92 = 17
   Nourished and identified not at risk, d, = 62.8% x 359 = 225
   Nourished and identified at risk, b, = 359-225 = 134
All frequencies a-d are greater than 10; hence formulae are valid.

For investigators with access to SPSS, Figure 8 presents SPSS commands which perform the sample size computations as outlined above. This requires the user to input values of prevalence, sensitivity and its maximum error of estimate, specificity and its maximum error into SPSS variables named *prev*, *sens*, *sensprec*, *spec* and *specprec* respectively. The SPSS routine can either be run by entering and running each line one by one in the Transform → IF and/or Compute option, or by entering all the commands in a SPSS syntax window and running them in one go. The required sample size figure for sensitivity is variable *senssize*, and for specificity the sample size is *specsize*. Using the smaller of these two values, the algorithm computes the expected frequencies *a* to *d* in the contingency table, to allow the user to check that these are greater than ten. Output using this routine on the data in Table 22 is given in Figure 9.

Establishment of Criterion Validity

As validity is a matter of degree and not an all-or-none property [91], an unqualified statement that criterion validity has been established should always be avoided. Evaluation of the criterion validity of a tool may well depend upon the choice of gold standard, and therefore it should always be reported in relation to that particular standard. The higher the values of sensitivity and specificity (or kappa), the more valid the tool is for this particular gold standard procedure.

Predictive Validity

Four of the 32 studies of a new tool and one of the 12 studies that either evaluated an existing tool in a new population or modified an existing instrument considered predictive validity. Details of the variables considered, assessment of independence of measures, number of subjects and method of analysis are presented in Tables 23(a) and 23(b), respectively, for each new tool, and for each existing or modified tool that had predictive validity assessed.

Variables

Predictive validity compares the tool with variables which will not be known until some time following application of the tool. For all but one study, the measures under consideration were considered constructs, as it would be expected that risk groups differ by these variables. Length of stay was a common variable for these studies. The remaining study [57] assessed predictive validity by comparing the tool with a subsequent criterion.

Independent Assessments

Only one study [44] stressed the independence of the information by using an investigator to abstract the required variables from patient's records, without knowledge of the tool's outcome and additional objective measurements. By using the same person to apply the nutritional screening tool and to collect the subsequent informatx³n, one study [57] introduced the possibility of bias.

Sample Size

The number of subjects ranged from 48 to 408; but no study justified its choice of sample size. Sample size determination for a numerical construct and for criterion validity were presented in previous sections of the book. Formulae to allow sample size calculation for a categorical variable are more complicated and hence it is suggested that statistical advice be sought.

Analysis

Standard techniques are required to compare the average value of a construct across the tool's risk groups, as outlined in the 'Analysis' part of the Construct Validity section. Length of stay was analysed using parametric tests, although none of the four studies reported that they had checked it followed an approximate normal distribution. Categorical variables, such as, post-operative complications and antibiotics usage, were appropriately analysed using a chi-square test. The level of agreement between the tool and the future gold standard was measured using specificity and sensitivity [57].

Case Summaries

PREV	SENS	SENSPREC	SPEC	SPECPREC	SENSSIZE	SPECSIZE	A	C	D	B
23.2	84.6	5	62.8	5	867	468	92	17	225	134

Figure 9. Output from SPSS routine (Figure 8) to calculate the sample size for a criterion validity study, using data from a published study [20]

Table 23(a). Studies that presented an original nutritional tool: Predictive validity

Population	Lead Author [Reference]	Variable	Independent[a] Assessments	Number of Subjects	Method of Analysis
Hospital Patients Adult	Ferguson [22]	Length of stay	Not stated	408	Analysis of variance
Hospital Patients Adult+Paediatric	Hunt [25]	Length of stay	Not stated	278	t test
Oral and Maxillo-facial Malignancy	Guo [39]	Post-operative complications Length of stay	Not stated	127	Chi-square test t test
Surgical	Baker [44]	Incidence of infection, antibiotics usage Length of stay	Yes	48	Chi-square test Analysis of variance

[a] Blinding of results from tool usage and future measurements

Table 23(b). Studies that evaluated an existing or modified nutritional tool: Predictive validity

Population	Lead Author [Reference]	Variable	Independent [a] Assessments	Number of Subjects	Method of Analysis
Medical and Surgical	Brown [57]	Subsequently received total parenteral nutrition or referral for dietary consultation	No	94	Specificity and sensitivity

[a] Blinding of results from tool usage and future measurements

REVIEW CONCLUSION

The review of published nutritional tools thus revealed that only a few studies evaluated predictive validity, and that this was primarily in relation to length of stay. As with construct and criterion validity, independent assessments, sample size and appropriate choice of statistical analysis were often overlooked.

Further Consideration of Validity

It would appear that an investigation to evaluate the validity of a nutritional screening or assessment tool may well require more subjects than that used by the majority of studies considered in the review. With possibly limited resources available to an investigator, this raises the question as to whether attention should be focused on a particular aspect of validity, which may have the most relevance for nutritional tool evaluation.

Most papers in the review evaluated a tool's validity with respect to variables recorded at a similar time to usage of the tool, and this would appear to be a more pertinent measure than a comparison with future features of a subject's prognosis. It would be anticipated that implementation of the screening programme would have a beneficial effect on a subject's care, with nutritional problems being identified and resolved earlier than if screening had not been implemented. This, in turn, would be expected to result in a shorter stay in hospital and a reduced incidence of subsequent adverse outcomes. Hence a comparison of such factors between the different risk categories of a tool is not confined to an evaluation of the tool's ability to discriminate between levels of risk but rather provides an overall assessment of the effectiveness of the subsequent plan of action to address potential or present nutritional problems. This clearly does not provide an evaluation of the tool's validity. Similarly, a comparison of the tool's outcome with subsequent referral for dietary consultation [57] merely audits the plan of dietary action.

As previously described, measurements made at a similar time to tool usage are either described as constructs or form a criterion. It is clearly germane to compare constructs, such as, nutritional parameters, anthropometric measurements and/or laboratory investigations between the risk categories of a tool, with the expectation that these would differ with the level of nutritional risk. However, the primary purpose of developing a nutritional screening or assessment tool is for it to aid the identification of subjects who are already malnourished or at risk of malnutrition. Hence it could be argued that the tool's ability to achieve this, as measured against a defined gold standard obtained at a similar time to the tool, leads to the most appropriate evaluation of the tool's validity.

A lack of consensus regarding an accepted gold standard is clearly a stumbling block. However, if a particular criterion has established psychometric properties in the intended subject population, based on sound methodological research, then it has gone a long way towards achieving scientific acceptance. There is, though, little to be gained in comparing a new instrument with an existing tool, for which little is known about its reliability and validity when applied in a similar population and under similar circumstances to those in which the new instrument will be used.

If a comparison of a tool with a chosen criterion results in a measure of validity which is not particularly high, this may be due to a number of factors. As already indicated, reliability places an upper limit on validity. To attempt to maximise the tool's reliability, it is important that the validity study is implemented in strict accordance with instructions regarding the tool's intended usage, and with the administrators of the tool receiving adequate training to help standardize their approach. In addition, there is the possibility that the criterion is not as reliable as had been anticipated. This may be a particular concern when the data arising from the criterion is subjectively evaluated. As previously discussed, a standardized procedure or repeat assessments by different experts may increase the reliability of the gold standard procedure.

Chapter 6

FURTHER APPLICATION OF FINDINGS

This book has presented criteria to aid a practitioner to assess the scientific merit of a nutritional screening or assessment tool using principles of sound design and analysis. The appraisal includes an assessment of the details regarding a tool's application, the methods used to derive the tool, and an evaluation of its performance. These features of a tool have been considered under the headings of application, development and evaluation. Specific criteria for assessing the quality of a tool and their rationale have been presented within each of these three sections, together with the results of applying these standards to published tools. Shortcomings identified by this review have been highlighted and the relevant methodology presented with examples of its application, to help ensure that future studies are implemented with regard to these important research principles. Practical suggestions have been made throughout to guide a practitioner as to the application of these findings.

The resultant critical appraisal of 44 published tools considered more features and additional detailed descriptions of tool methodology than it was possible to include in the original review [13]. The conclusion of this previous study was that not one tool was judged to have satisfied a set of criteria regarding scientific merit. This raises the questions as to what, if anything, can be salvaged from this seemingly hopeless situation?

If the error is one of omission of details from a publication, then this may be less serious than that of a poor quality investigation. Absence of information relating to a tool's application places the onus on potential users of the tool to contact the authors to obtain the missing information which will allow the instrument to be correctly applied.

The omission of an exhaustive evidence base for a tool's content suggests that this tool is best avoided. An apparent lack of scientific rigour in the development process of a tool clearly casts doubt on its potential value. Measures of a tool's reliability and validity, if based on well designed studies, will be a key factor influencing the decision of practitioners to proceed with this instrument.

Although an existing instrument may have limitations, this does not necessarily warrant the development of a new tool. In some situations, it may be possible to adapt an existing tool and then assess the suitability and performance of the modified version. For example, it may be desirable to adapt a tool, developed for use by a particular professional group, to make it more suitable for a different group of users.

However, if no relevant tool exists for an intended population, or the deficiencies of existing instruments severely limit their value, then there is justification for the development of a new instrument. However, as is evident from this book, the derivation and subsequent evaluation of a tool involves a considerable amount of time and effort, and is likely to require larger studies than that used previously. Hence there must be strong evidence for the need of another tool, and this would form the basis for the submission to the local research ethics committee and to funding bodies [59].

Tools for assessment of malnutrition continue to be developed and published. The development of some of these was justified on the grounds that no relevant tool existed for a particular group of subjects. For example, the Nutrition Risk Score [23] has been adapted for use amongst mental health clients [95], and Mackintosh and Hankey [96] developed a tool for elderly patients attending community day hospitals because such a validated tool was unavailable. Despite the presence of several tools for use amongst hospital in-patients, new ones continue to be published, with no explanation of why existing instruments are inappropriate [97,98].

Of particular note is a malnutrition screening tool published by the Malnutrition Advisory Group (MAG), a standing committee of the British Association for Parenteral and Enteral Nutrition (BAPEN). This tool was developed by a multi-disciplinary group, with the initial purpose to detect and manage under-nutrition in adults in the community. The original tool has now been extended for use in various health care settings and by all care workers, and is termed the Malnutrition Universal Screening Tool ('MUST'). It categorises subjects into low, medium, or high risk of malnutrition and identifies the obese. The tool involves assessment of BMI, unintentional weight loss in the previous three to six months and the presence of an acute disease resulting in no dietary intake for more than five days. The tool and an explanatory booklet, which contains guidance for its usage and taking measurements, as well as management guidelines for developing care plans, can be downloaded from the BAPEN website [99]. It has been shown to be quick and easy to use [100].

The 'MUST' tool is the first universal screening tool, designed for the whole health care spectrum, and for use by different health care professionals and different patient groups [101]. Others have suggested that a generic nutritional instrument (with reference only to in-patients) is preferable to one developed for use in a specific population [21-23]. However, the appropriateness of a generic tool depends upon whether the important factors associated with nutritional risk are common across all subjects in the intended population. If the risk factors are not specific enough for particular subgroups of individuals, the ability of the screening tool to detect malnutrition will be reduced.

It is regrettable that the 'MUST' report [102], which details the tool's development and results of reliability and validity studies, is not freely available. This restricts the opportunity for practitioners to appraise the scientific meritoriousness of the instrument using criteria presented in this book. As the report is not in stock at the British Library, the author has not yet accessed this information. A recently published study [100] of the tool's criterion validity when compared to seven other screening tools concluded that there was fair-good to excellent agreement beyond chance. However, such a comparison with tools, some of which lack evidence of established psychometric properties, limits the value of this assessment.

The ability to implement the same tool to screen subjects as they move from one healthcare setting to another is a definite advantage. If the 'MUST' has been rigorously developed, and proves to be reliable and valid based on well designed investigations, when used in all health care settings by various administrators, then this will be a deciding factor in determining its acceptance as a universal screening tool.

Guidelines [6] from the European Society of Parenteral and Enteral Nutrition (ESPEN) currently recommend three different tools for screening adults: 'MUST' for use in the community, Nutrition Risk Screening (NRS-2002) in hospital, and the Mini Nutritional Assessment (MNA) for the elderly. Copies of these tools are included with the guidelines [6]. In addition to the nutritional components of 'MUST', the NRS-2002 [103] also contains a grading of severity of disease. The MNA is a shortened version of the original tool for use amongst the elderly [18]. It has though, been acknowledged [6], that the present recommendations by ESPEN may share some of the short-comings identified by the author's evaluation [13] of the scientific credibility of nutritional tools. It was therefore concluded that these recommendations may need to be modified in the light of future experience.

CONCLUSION

The large number of nutritional screening and assessment tools in existence indicates that a substantial amount of time, effort and resources has been expended on developing these instruments to assist in the diagnosis of malnutrition. Unfortunately, this process has invariably overlooked the vital importance of carrying out this research using principles of good design and analysis.

Criteria for assessing the scientific merit of a tool were applied to an array of 44 published tools. Each tool was assessed in relation to details of its application, method of derivation and evaluation of its performance. The fact that authors of many tools did not publish full details regarding its intended usage makes it impossible for potential users to know whether they are correctly applying the tool. An apparent lack of scientific rigour in the development of some of the tools casts doubt on their value and usefulness. In particular, the majority of tools based on a sum of scores approach, appeared to use an arbitrary scoring system, and hence overlooked the importance of this critical aspect of tool development. This suggests that a unified approach using a multivariate analysis could play an important role in the development of future nutritional screening and assessment tools. The performance of many tools, as measured by their reliability and validity, has not been assessed. Those which have implemented reliability and validity studies have given inadequate attention to important design issues, such as, independent assessments, use of appropriate administrators and adequate sample size. This coupled with incorrect methods of analysis will not provide informative estimates oV%a tool's performance.

There is clearly a need to ensure that nutritional screening and assessment tools are developed using procedures based on sound methodological principles. Developers of a tool have an ethical responsibility to provide comprehensive instructions for its usage, evidence of a scientific basis to its derivation and composition, and confirmation that it performs well. Otherwise a tool may be little more than worthless pieces of paper, the completion of which wastes time and resources. Moreover, such a tool will not provide useful data, resulting in the likely misclassification of nutritional risk and hence could have serious consequences to patient care.

REFERENCES

[1] McWhirter, JP; Pennington, CR. Incidence and recognition of malnutrition in hospital. *BMJ*, 1994; 308, 945-948.

[2] Chima, CS; Barco, K; Dewitt, MLA; Maeda, M; Teran, JC; Mullen, KD. Relationship of nutritional status to length of stay, hospital costs, and discharge status of patients hospitalized in the medicine service. *J. Am. Diet Assoc*, 1997; 97, 975-978.

[3] Lennard-Jones, JE. A positive approach to nutrition as treatment: A report of a working party on the role of enteral and parenteral feeding in hospital and at home. London: King's Fund Centre; 1992.

[4] Silk, DBA. *Organisation of nutritional support in hospitals*. A report by a working party of the British Association for Parenteral and Enteral Nutrition. Kent: BAPEN; 1994.

[5] Kushner, RF; Ayello, EA; Beyer, PL; Skipper, A; Van Way, CW; Young, EA; Balogun, LB. National Coordinating Committee clinical indicators of nutrition care. *J. Am. Diet Assoc*, 1994; 94, 1168-1177.

[6] Kondrup, J; Allison, SP; Elia, M; Vellas, B; Plauth, M. ESPEN guidelines for nutrition screening 2002. *Clin. Nutr,* 2003; 22, 415-421.

[7] McLaren, S; Holmes, S; Green, S; Bond, S. An overview of nutritional issues relating to the care of older people in hospital. In: Bond S, editor. *Eating matters: A resource for improving dietary care in hospitals*. Newcastle upon Tyne: University of Newcastle upon Tyne Press; 1997; 15-100.

[8] Holmes, S. Nutritional screening and older adults. *Nurs. Stand*, 2000; 15, 42-44.

[9] Green, SM; McLaren, SG. Nutritional assessment and screening: instrument selection. *Br. J. Community Nurs*, 1998; 3, 233-242.

[10] Arrowsmith, H. A critical evaluation of the use of nutrition screening tools by nurses. *Br. J. Nurs*, 1999; 8, 1483-1490.
[11] Lyne, PA; Prowse, MA. Methodological issues in the development and use of instruments to assess patient nutritional status or the level of risk of nutritional compromise. *J. Adv. Nurs*, 1999; 30, 835-842.
[12] Laporte, M; Villalon, L; Payette, H. Simple nutrition screening tools for healthcare facilities: development and validity assessment. *Canad. J. Diet Pract. Res*, 2001; 62, 26-34.
[13] Jones, JM. The methodology of nutritional screening and assessment tools. *J. Hum. Nutr. Dietet*, 2002; 15, 59-71.
[14] Clark, MP; Oakland, MJ; Brotherson, MJ. Nutrition screening for children with special health care needs. *Children's Health Care*, 1998; 27, 231-245.
[15] Campbell, MK; Kelsey, KS. The PEACH survey: A nutrition screening tool for use in early intervention programs. *J. Am. Diet Assoc*, 1994; 94, 1156-1158.
[16] Gilford, A; Khun Khun, R. Development of nutritional risk screening in the community. *British Journal of Community Health Nursing*, 1996; 1, 335-336,338-339.
[17] Ward, J; Close, J; Little, J; Boorman, J; Perkins, A; Coles, SJ; Edington, JD. Development of a screening tool for assessing risk of undernutrition in patients in the community. *J. Hum. Nutr. Dietet*, 1998; 11, 323-330.
[18] Guigoz, Y; Vellas, B; Garry, PJ. Assessing the nutritional status of the elderly: The Mini Nutritional Assessment as part of the geriatric evaluation. *Nutr. Rev*, 1996; 54, S59-S65.
[19] Wolinsky, FD; Coe, RM; McIntosh, WA; Kubena, KS; Prendergast, JM; Chavez, MN; Miller, DK; Romeis, JC; Landmann, WA. Progress in the development of a Nutritional Risk Index. *J. Nutr*, 1990; 120, 1549-1553.
[20] Kovacevich, DS; Boney, AR; Braunschweig, CL; Perez, A; Stevens, M. Nutrition risk classification: A reproducible and valid tool for nurses. *Nutr. Clin. Pract*, 1997; 12, 20-25.
[21] Goudge, DR; Williams, A; Pinnington, LL. Development, validity and reliability of the Derby Nutritional Score. *J. Hum. Nutr. Dietet*, 1998; 11, 411-421.
[22] Ferguson, M; Capra, S; Bauer, J; Banks, M. Development of a valid and reliable malnutrition screening tool for adult acute hospital patients. *Nutrition*, 1999; 15, 458-464.

[23] Reilly, HM; Martineau, JK; Moran, A; Kennedy, H. Nutritional screening - Evaluation and implementation of a simple Nutrition Risk Score. *Clin. Nutr*, 1995; 14, 269-273.
[24] Nagel, MR. Nutrition screening: Identifying patients at risk for malnutrition. *Nutr. Clin. Pract*, 1993; 8, 171-175.
[25] Hunt, DR; Maslovitz, A; Rowlands, BJ; Brooks, B. A simple nutrition screening procedure for hospital patients. *J. Am. Diet. Assoc*, 1985; 85, 332-335.
[26] Hedberg, A-M; Garcia, N; Trejus, IJ; Weinmann-Winkler, S; Gabriel, ML; Lutz, AL. Nutritional risk screening: Development of a standardized protocol using dietetic technicians. *J. Am. Diet. Assoc*, 1988; 88, 1553-1556.
[27] Lowery, JC; Hiller, LD; Davis, JA; Shore, CJ. Comparison of professional judgment versus an algorithm for nutrition status classification. *Med. Care*, 1998; 36, 1578-1588.
[28] Pattison, R; Corr, J; Ogilvie, M; Farquhar, D; Sutherland, D; Davidson, HIM; Richardson, RA. Reliability of a qualitative screening tool versus physical measurements in identifying undernutrition in an elderly population. *J. Hum. Nutr. Dietet,* 1999; 12, 133-140.
[29] Cotton, E; Zinober, B; Jessop, J. A nutritional assessment tool for older patients. *Prof. Nurse*, 1996; 11, 609-610,612.
[30] Nikolaus, T; Bach, M; Siezen, S; Volkert, D; Oster, P; Schlierf, G. Assessment of nutritional risk in the elderly. *Ann. Nutr. Metab*, 1995; 39, 340-345.
[31] Henderson, CJ; Lovell, DJ; Gregg, DJ. A nutritional screening test for use in children and adolescents with juvenile rheumatoid arthritis. *J. Rheumatol*, 1992; 19, 1276-1281.
[32] Bryan, F; Jones, JM; Russell, L. Reliability and validity of a nutrition screening tool to be used with clients with learning difficulties. *J. Hum. Nutr. Dietet*, 1998; 11, 41-50.
[33] Noel, MB; Wojnaroski, SM. Nutrition screening for long-term care residents. *J. Am. Diet. Assoc*, 1987; 87, 1557-1558.
[34] Potosnak, L; Chudnow, LP; Simko, MD. A simple tool for identifying patients at nutritional risk. *Qual. Rev. Bull*, 1983; 9, 81-83.
[35] Oakley, C; Hill, R. Nutrition assessment score validation and the implications for usage. *J. Hum. Nutr. Dietet*, 2000; 13, 343-352.
[36] Elmore, MF; Wagner, DR; Knoll, DM; Eizember, L; Oswalt, MA; Glowinski, EA; Rapp, PA. Developing an effective adult nutrition screening tool for a community hospital. *J. Am. Diet. Assoc*, 1994; 94, 1113-1118,1121.

[37] Lundvick, J; Phillips, R. Nutritional screening of the oncology patient. *Nutr. Support Serv*, 1983; 3, 21,23-24.
[38] Latkany, L; Lloyd, ME; Schaeffer, A. Development of adult and pediatric oncology nutrition screening tools. *Top Clin. Nutr*, 1995; 10, 85-89.
[39] Guo, C-B; Ma, D-Q; Zhang K-H. Applicability of the general nutritional status score to patients with oral and maxillofacial malignancies. *Int. J. Oral Maxillofac Surg*, 1994; 23, 167-169.
[40] Hall, JC; Yap, L. The assessment of nutritional status in surgical patients. *Aust. Clin. Rev*, 1987; 7, 175-177.
[41] Lupo, L; Pannarale, O; Altomare, D; Memeo, V; Rubino, M. Reliability of clinical judgement in evaluation of the nutritional status of surgical patients. *Br. J. Surg*, 1993; 80, 1553-1556.
[42] Scanlan, F; Dunne, J; Toyne, K. No more cause for neglect. Introducing a nutritional assessment tool and action plan. *Prof. Nurse*, 1994; 9, 382,384-385.
[43] Thompson, JS; Burrough, CA; Green, JL; Brown, GL. Nutritional screening in surgical patients. *J. Am. Diet. Assoc*, 1984; 84, 337-338.
[44] Baker, JP; Detsky, AS; Wesson, DE; Wolman, SL; Stewart, S; Whitewell, J; Langer, B; Jeejeebhoy, KN. Nutritional assessment: A comparison of clinical judgement and objective measurements. *N. Engl. J. Med*, 1982; 306, 969-972.
[45] Cooper, N. Audit in clinical practice: evaluating use of a nutrition screening tool developed for trauma nurses. *J. Hum. Nutr. Dietet*, 1988; 11, 403-410.
[46] Hickson, M; Hill, M. Implementing a nutritional assessment tool in the community: a report describing the process, audit and problems encountered. *J. Hum. Nutr. Dietet*, 1997; 10, 373-377.
[47] Kalantar-Zadeh, K; Kleiner, M; Dunne, E; Lee, GH; Luft, FC. A modified quantitative subjective global assessment of nutrition for dialysis patients. *Nephrol. Dial. Transplant*, 1999; 14, 1732-1738.
[48] Enia G, Sicuso C, Alati G, Zoccali C. Subjective global assessment of nutrition in dialysis patients, *Nephrol. Dial. Transplant,* 1993; 8, 1094-1098
[49] Visser, R; Dekker, FW; Boeschoten, EW; Stevens, P; Krediet, RT. Reliability of the 7-point subjective global assessment scale in assessing nutritional status of dialysis patients. *Adv. Perit. Dial*, 1999; 15, 222-225.

[50] Ek, A-C; Unosson, M; Larsson, J; Ganowiak, W; Bjurulf, P. Interrater variability and validity in subjective nutritional assessment of elderly patients. *Scand. J. Caring. Sci*, 1996; 10, 163-168.

[51] Prendergast, JM; Coe, RM; Chavez, MN; Romeis, JC; Miller, DK; Wolinsky, FD. Clinical validation of a nutritional risk index. *J. Community Health*, 1989; 14, 125-135.

[52] Wright, L. A nutritional screening tool for use by nurses in residential and nursing homes for elderly people: development and pilot study results. *J. Hum. Nutr. Dietet*, 1999; 12, 437-443.

[53] Detsky, AS; McLaughlin, JR; Baker, JP; Johnston, N; Whittaker, S; Mendelson, RA; Jeejeebhoy, KN. What is subjective global assessment of nutritional status?. *JPEN*, 1987; 11, 8-13.

[54] Hirsch, S; de Obaldia, N; Petermann, M; Rojo, P; Barrientos, C; Iturriaga, H; Bunout, D. Subjective global assessment of nutritional status: Further validation. *Nutrition*, 1991; 7, 35-37.

[55] Bowers, JM; Dols, CL. Subjective global assessment in HIV-infected patients. *J. Assoc. Nurses AIDS Care*, 1996; 7, 83-89.

[56] Hasse, J; Strong, S; Gorman, MA; Liepa, G. Subjective global assessment: Alternative nutrition-assessment technique for liver-transplant candidates. *Nutrition*, 1993; 9, 339-343.

[57] Brown, CSB; Stegman, MR. Nutritional assessment of surgical patients. *Qual. Rev. Bull*, 1988; 14, 302-306.

[58] Foltz, MB; Schiller, MR; Ryan, AS. Nutrition screening and assessment: Current practices and dietitians' leadership roles. *J. Am. Diet. Assoc*, 1993; 93, 1388-1395.

[59] Jones, JM. Development of a nutritional screening or assessment tool using a multivariate technique. *Nutrition*, 2004; 20, 298-306.

[60] Sizer, T. Standards and guidelines for nutritional support of patients in hospitals. A report by a working party of the British Association for Parenteral and Enteral Nutrition. Maidenhead: BAPEN; 1996.

[61] McLaren, S; Green, S. Nutritional screening and assessment. *Prof. Nurse. Study Suppl*, 1998; 13, S9-S15.

[62] Edington, J. Problems of nutritional assessment in the community. *Proc.. Nutr. Soc*, 1999; 58, 47-51.

[63] Oppenheim, AN. Questionnaire design, interviewing and attitude measurement. London: Pinter Publishers; 1992.

[64] Jones, JM; Maryosh, J; Johnstone, S; Templeton, J. A multivariate analysis of factors related to the mortality of blunt trauma admissions to the North Staffordshire Hospital Centre. *J. Trauma*, 1995; 38, 118-122.

[65] Potter, RG; Jones, JM; Boardman, AP. A prospective study of primary care patients with musculoskeletal pain: the identification of predictive factors for chronicity. *Br. J. Gen. Pract*, 2000; 50, 225-227.
[66] MacKintosh, JF; Cowan, RA; Jones, M; Harris, M; Deakin, DP; Crowther, D. Prognostic factors in stage I and II high and intermediate grade non-Hodgkin's lymphoma. *Eur. J. Cancer Clin. Oncol*, 1988; 24, 1617-1622.
[67] Deeks, JJ. Systematic reviews of evaluations of diagnostic and screening tests. *BMJ*, 2001; 323, 157-162.
[68] Harrell, FE; Lee, KL; Mark, DB. Multivariable prognostic models: Issues in developing models, evaluating assumptions and adequacy, and measuring and reducing errors. *Statist. Med*, 1996; 15, 361-387.
[69] Hosmer, DW; Lemeshow, S. Applied logistic regression. New York: Wiley; 2000.
[70] SPSS Inc. SPSS for Windows, release 11. Chicago: SPSS Inc.; 2001.
[71] Minitab Inc. Minitab for Windows, release 13. State College: Minitab Inc.; 2000.
[72] Jones, JM. Uses and abuses of statistical models for evaluating trauma care. *J. Trauma*, 1995; 38, 89-93.
[73] Lee, ET. Statistical methods for survival data analysis. Belmont: Lifetime Learning Publications; 1980.
[74] Kline, P. An easy guide to factor analysis. London: Routledge; 1994.
[75] Streiner, DL; Norman, GR. Health measurement scales. A practical guide to their development and use. 2nd edition. Oxford: Oxford University Press; 1995.
[76] Cronbach, LJ. Coefficient alpha and the internal structure of tests. *Psychometrika*, 1951; 16, 297-334.
[77] Dunn, G. Design and analysis of reliability studies: The statistical evaluation of measurement errors. London: Edward Arnold; 1992.
[78] Jones, JM. Reliability of nutritional screening and assessment tools. *Nutrition*, 2004; 20, 307-311.
[79] Altaye, M; Donner, A; Eliasziw, M. A general goodness-of-fit approach for inference procedures concerning the kappa statistic. *Statist. Med*, 2001; 20, 2479-2488.
[80] Cohen, J. A coefficient of agreement for nominal scales. *Educ. Psychol. Meas*, 1960; 20, 37-46.
[81] Landis, JR; Koch, GG. The measurement of observer agreement for categorical data. *Biometrics*, 1977; 33, 159-174.
[82] Shrout, PE. Measurement reliability and agreement in psychiatry. *Statist. Methods Med. Res*, 1998; 7, 301-317.

[83] Fleiss, JL; Cohen, J; Everitt, BS. Large sample standard errors of kappa and weighted kappa. *Psychol. Bull*, 1969; 72, 323-327.
[84] Cantor, AB. Sample size calculations for Cohen's Kappa. *Psychol. Methods*, 1996; 1, 150-153.
[85] Donner, A; Eliasziw, M. A goodness-of-fit approach to inference procedures for the kappa statistic: Confidence interval construction, significance-testing and sample size estimation. *Statist. Med*, 1992; 11, 1511-1519.
[86] Flack, VF; Afifi, AA; Lachenbruch, PA; Schouten, HJA. Sample size determinations for the two rater kappa statistic. *Psychometrika*, 1988; 53, 321-325.
[87] Altman, DG. Practical statistics for medical research. London: Chapman and Hall; 1991.
[88] Streiner, DL. Learning how to differ: Agreement and reliability statistics in psychiatry. *Can. J. Psychiatry*, 1995; 40, 60-66.
[89] Haas, M. Statistical methodology for reliability studies. *J. Manipulative Physiol. Ther*, 1991; 14, 119-132.
[90] Shrout, PE; Fleiss, JL. Intraclass correlations: Uses in assessing rater reliability. *Psychol. Bull*, 1979; 86, 420-428.
[91] Carmines, EG; Zeller, RA. Reliability and validity assessment. In: Lewis-Beck MS, editor. *Basic measurement*. London: Sage Publications; 1994; 1-58.
[92] Morley, S; Snaith, P. Principles of psychological assessment. In: Freeman C, Tyrer P, editors. *Research methods in psychiatry: a beginner's guide*. 2nd edition. London: Gaskell; 1992; 135-152.
[93] Jones, JM. Validity of nutritional screening and assessment tools. *Nutrition*, 2004; 20, 312-317.
[94] Cohen, J. Statistical power analysis for the behavioural sciences. 2nd edition. New Jersey: Lawrence Erlbaum Associates; 1988.
[95] Abayomi, J; Hackett, A. Assessment of malnutrition in mental health clients: nurses' judgement vs. a nutrition risk tool. *J. Adv. Nurs*, 2004; 45, 430-437.
[96] Mackintosh, MA; Hankey, CR. Reliability of a nutrition screening tool for use in elderly day hospitals. *J. Hum. Nutr. Diet*, 2001; 14, 129-136.
[97] Burden, ST; Bodey, S; Bradburn, YJ; Murdoch, S; Thompson, AL; Sim, JM; Sowerbutts, AM. Validation of a nutrition screening tool: testing the reliability and validity. *J. Hum. Nutr. Diet*, 2001; 14, 269-275.
[98] Doyle, MP; Barnes, E; Moloney, M. The evaluation of an undernutrition risk score to be used by nursing staff in a teaching

hospital to identify surgical patients at risk of malnutrition on admission: a pilot study. *J. Hum. Nutr. Diet*, 2000; 13, 433-441.

[99] 'Malnutrition Universal Screening Tool' (The 'MUST'). Available from http://bapen.org.uk/the-must.htm.

[100] Stratton, RJ; Hackston, A; Longmore, D; Dixon, R; Price, S; Stroud, M; King, C; Elia, M. Malnutrition in hospital outpatients and inpatients: prevalence, concurrent validity and ease of use of the 'malnutrition universal screening tool' ('MUST') for adults. *Br. J. Nutr*, 2004; 92, 799-808.

[101] Malnutrition Advisory Group. A consistent and reliable tool for malnutrition screening. *Nurs. Times*, 2003; 99, 26-27.

[102] Elia, M. Screening for malnutrition: A multidisciplinary responsibility. Development and use of the 'malnutrition universal screening tool' ('MUST') for adults. A report by the Malnutrition Advisory Group, a standing committee of BAPEN. Worcs.: BAPEN; 2003.

[103] Kondrup, J; Rasmussen, HH; Hamberg, O; Stanga, Z. Nutritional risk screening (NRS 2002): A new method based on an analysis of controlled clinical trials. *Clin. Nutr*, 2003; 22, 321-336.

INDEX

A

acceptance, 85, 89
access, 44, 68, 80
accuracy, 38, 43, 76
adjustment, 68
administrators, vii, 5, 7, 13, 14, 34, 37, 39, 57, 58, 61, 85, 89, 91
adolescents, 95
adults, 88, 89, 100
age, 8, 27
AIDS, 97
albumin, 71
algorithm, 16, 18, 19, 20, 32, 50, 80, 95
alternative, 29, 48, 61, 76
ambiguity, 52
assessment, vii, ix, x, 1, 2, 8, 9, 10, 12, 16, 17, 21, 24, 30, 31, 32, 33, 34, 37, 40, 55, 56, 58, 61, 62, 63, 65, 70, 71, 72, 73, 75, 78, 81, 84, 87, 88, 89, 91, 93, 94, 95, 96, 97, 98, 99
assessment tools, vii, ix, x, 2, 21, 33, 91, 94, 98, 99
association, 16, 24, 39, 76
assumptions, 39, 98
attention, 13, 39, 62, 66, 84, 91
availability, x, 5, 14

B

beneficial effect, 84
bias, 15, 24, 33, 81
BMI, 26, 27, 28, 88
body, 2, 26, 62
body mass index, 2, 26, 62

C

candidates, 97
children, 94, 95
classification, 23, 29, 42, 52, 94, 95
clients, 88, 95, 99
clinical trials, 100
cohort, 24
community, ix, 2, 25, 68, 88, 89, 94, 95, 96, 97
compilation, 14
complications, 81, 82
components, 89
composition, 32, 92
computation, 32
concentrates, 33
confidence, 32, 34, 38, 42, 43, 44, 45, 46, 47, 50, 51, 52, 75, 77, 79
confidence interval, 34, 38, 42, 43, 44, 45, 46, 47, 50, 51, 52, 75, 77, 79
consensus, 31, 70, 74, 85

construct validity, 55, 56, 62, 65, 66, 67, 68, 69, 70
consumption, 8
contamination, 74
context, 5, 44, 52, 65, 67
contingency, 79, 80
cooking, 28
correlation, 32, 35, 36, 39, 51, 52, 63, 64, 65, 71
correlation analysis, 65
costs, 93
credibility, 90

D

data analysis, 98
database, 29, 46, 50, 69, 79
decisions, 52
definition, 7, 8, 13, 66, 70, 74
deviation, 67, 68
dialysis, 96
dietary intake, 88
disabilities, 25
discordance, 74
discriminant analysis, 16, 31
discrimination, 25, 29
distribution, 44, 65

E

elderly, ix, 88, 89, 94, 95, 97, 99
environment, ix
estimating, 23, 38, 76
ethics, 88
evidence, x, 5, 13, 14, 30, 32, 88, 89, 92
exclusion, 7, 27
expectation, 84
expertise, 14, 37, 61
experts, 55, 74, 85
exposure, x

F

face validity, 31

factor analysis, 31, 98
family, 9
feedback, 15
food, 8
friends, 9
funding, 88

G

generation, 29
gold, 16, 20, 24, 25, 31, 55, 56, 57, 70, 72, 73, 74, 75, 76, 80, 81, 85
grades, 20
grading, 89
groups, ix, 1, 7, 8, 12, 13, 17, 19, 20, 21, 24, 25, 26, 29, 30, 31, 34, 37, 48, 58, 64, 65, 66, 67, 68, 69, 70, 74, 75, 81, 89
guidance, x, 89
guidelines, vii, ix, x, 16, 89, 93, 97

H

health, vii, ix, 9, 10, 12, 13, 17, 88, 89, 94
health care, vii, ix, 9, 10, 12, 88, 89, 94
health care professionals, 10, 89
health services, 17
health status, 17
HIV, 4, 12, 19, 60, 64, 97
hypothesis, 67, 70
hypothesis test, 67

I

identification, vii, ix, x, 21, 24, 27, 84, 98
implementation, 7, 43, 52, 53, 62, 77, 84, 95
incidence, 84
inclusion, 7, 8, 26, 27
independence, vii, 34, 62, 70, 74, 81
indication, 32, 33, 37, 58
indicators, 16, 23, 28, 31, 93

industry, ix
infection, 82
influence, 50
input, 44, 50, 68, 80
instruction, 15
instruments, x, 1, 14, 17, 33, 56, 70, 88, 91, 94
interest, 5, 52, 65
internal consistency, 31
interpretation, 43, 47, 74, 75
interval, 33, 42, 43, 44, 77, 79, 99
intervention, 9, 94

J

judges, 20
judgment, 14, 95
justification, 14, 17, 20, 66, 88
juvenile rheumatoid arthritis, 95

K

knowledge, 32, 65, 81

L

lead, 38
leadership, 97
learning, 95
learning difficulties, 95
likelihood, 27
limitation, 31, 44
liver, 12
liver transplant, 12
low risk, 31, 73
lymphoma, 98

M

Mackintosh, 88, 99
malnutrition, vii, ix, x, 1, 2, 5, 11, 12, 13, 14, 15, 16, 19, 20, 21, 23, 24, 25, 26, 27, 28, 29, 30, 31, 32, 43, 51, 55, 65, 66, 67, 68, 70, 77, 78, 85, 88, 89, 91, 93, 94, 95, 99, 100
management, 48, 89
mass, 26, 28
meals, 8
measurement, 29, 51, 52, 97, 98, 99
measures, 29, 31, 33, 39, 52, 55, 56, 63, 64, 70, 75, 81
memory, 33
mental health, 88, 99
methodology, vii, x, 1, 7, 27, 32, 34, 39, 56, 66, 76, 87, 94, 99
models, 21, 98
monitoring, 8
morbidity, vii, ix
mortality, vii, ix, 97
multiple regression, 16, 20, 31
multiple regression analyses, 16
multiple regression analysis, 31

N

needs, 5, 12, 15, 28, 66
normal distribution, 31, 65, 66, 67, 69, 81
nurses, 13, 35, 37, 59, 61, 94, 96, 97, 99
nursing, 2, 8, 9, 73, 97, 99
nutritional assessment, x, 11, 40, 63, 64, 70, 73, 74, 95, 96, 97
nutritional screening, vii, ix, x, 1, 2, 16, 21, 28, 29, 33, 65, 70, 74, 81, 84, 87, 91, 94, 95, 97, 98, 99

O

objective criteria, 42
older adults, 93
older people, 93
omission, 87, 88
ordinal data, 39, 47, 48, 50, 52
outline, 21

Index

P

pain, 98
parameter, 32, 66
parameter estimates, 32
peritoneum, 12
perspective, 26
pilot study, 14, 15, 25, 43, 53, 77, 97, 100
poor, 87
population, vii, ix, x, 1, 2, 5, 7, 8, 13, 14, 17, 24, 25, 30, 34, 38, 43, 50, 56, 57, 58, 62, 67, 68, 70, 76, 77, 80, 85, 88, 89, 95
power, 67, 69, 99
predictive validity, 55, 80, 81, 84
predictors, 14, 16, 31
preference, 16
probability, 23, 27, 29, 30, 38, 66, 67
production, ix, 15
prognosis, 84
program, 29
protocol, 29, 34, 56, 70, 71, 95
psychometric properties, 85, 89

R

range, 8, 19, 20, 42, 43, 44
reasoning, 19, 66
recall, 33
recognition, 93
recovery, vii, ix
recruiting, 77
reduction, 16
reflection, 76
regression, 17, 21, 27, 30, 31, 32, 98
regression analysis, 17, 27, 31, 32
regression method, 31
relationship, 20, 25, 26
relationships, 62
relevance, 14, 33, 55, 84
reliability, vii, 24, 32, 33, 34, 37, 38, 39, 40, 42, 43, 44, 45, 46, 47, 48, 50, 51, 52, 53, 56, 61, 74, 85, 88, 89, 91, 94, 98, 99
resources, 32, 38, 84, 91, 92
responsibility, 32, 92, 100
risk, vii, ix, x, 1, 5, 7, 8, 9, 10, 11, 12, 14, 15, 16, 17, 19, 20, 23, 24, 25, 26, 27, 28, 29, 30, 31, 32, 39, 40, 41, 44, 45, 46, 47, 50, 51, 52, 55, 61, 62, 64, 65, 66, 67, 68, 69, 70, 71, 72, 73, 74, 75, 78, 80, 81, 84, 88, 89, 92, 94, 95, 97, 99, 100
risk factors, ix, 14, 16, 17, 23, 24, 25, 27, 29, 31, 89
routines, vii

S

sample, vii, 25, 34, 38, 39, 43, 44, 46, 47, 50, 51, 57, 58, 65, 66, 67, 68, 69, 76, 77, 78, 79, 80, 81, 82, 84, 91, 99
sampling, 24, 34, 58
scores, 16, 18, 19, 20, 23, 24, 26, 27, 51, 52, 91
search, 1, 2, 5, 7, 13, 14
selecting, 27
sensitivity, 16, 20, 29, 71, 72, 75, 76, 77, 78, 79, 80, 81, 83
series, 17
severity, 17, 89
shares, 42
significance level, 67, 68, 69
skills, 13
specificity, 16, 20, 29, 75, 76, 77, 78, 79, 80, 81
spectrum, 89
SPSS, vii, 27, 44, 46, 47, 50, 51, 68, 69, 79, 80, 82, 98
stages, 5
standard deviation, 67, 68
standard error, 32, 38, 41, 42, 44, 50, 99
standards, vii, 56, 87
statistics, 99
stock, 89
strength, 20, 44

survival, 98
systems, 20, 48

T

teaching, 99
technician, 9
time, 2, 5, 7, 8, 9, 12, 14, 15, 29, 30, 32, 33, 38, 56, 62, 81, 84, 88, 91, 92
time frame, 14
total parenteral nutrition, 83
training, 5, 15, 37, 52, 53, 61, 85
trauma, 96, 97, 98
trial, 16
triceps, 66, 67, 68, 69

U

UK, viii, ix
undernutrition, 94, 95, 99
uniform, 21

V

validation, 30, 95, 97
validity, vii, 14, 15, 32, 55, 56, 57, 58, 59, 60, 61, 62, 63, 64, 65, 66, 68, 69, 70, 71, 72, 73, 74, 75, 76, 77, 78, 79, 80, 81, 82, 83, 84, 85, 88, 89, 91, 94, 95, 97, 99, 100
values, 26, 27, 29, 42, 44, 50, 61, 63, 68, 76, 78, 80
variability, 51, 97
variable, 1, 7, 8, 9, 12, 14, 17, 19, 20, 24, 25, 26, 27, 31, 32, 39, 40, 42, 43, 45, 46, 47, 48, 50, 55, 56, 65, 66, 67, 68, 69, 70, 79, 80, 81
variables, ix, 14, 15, 16, 17, 18, 19, 20, 23, 24, 25, 26, 27, 30, 31, 32, 44, 46, 50, 51, 55, 56, 62, 65, 66, 68, 69, 70, 79, 80, 81, 84
variance, 51, 63, 64, 65, 66, 67, 69, 82
variation, 67

W

weight loss, 88
work, 32, 33, 37, 39, 56, 62
workers, 88

Y

yes/no, 17
yield, 37, 61